Milady's Standard Esthetics: Fundamentals Exam Review

Tenth Edition

Jeryl Spear

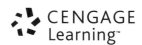
CENGAGE
Learning™

Australia • Brazil • Japan • Korea • Mexico • Singapore • Spain • United Kingdom • United States

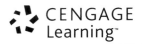
CENGAGE
Learning™

Milady's Standard Esthetics: Fundamentals Exam Review, Tenth Edition

Jeryl Spear

President, Milady: Dawn Gerrain

Publisher: Erin O'Connor

Acquisitions Editor: Martine Edwards

Product Manager: Jessica Burns

Editorial Assistant: Mike Spring

Director of Beauty Industry Relations: Sandra Bruce

Senior Marketing Manager: Gerard McAvey

Marketing Specialist: Erica Conley

Production Director: Wendy Troeger

Senior Content Project Manager: Nina Tucciarelli

Art Director: Joy Kocsis

For product information and technology assistance, contact us at
Professional & Career Group Customer Support, 1-800-648-7450

For permission to use material from this text or product, submit all requests online at **cengage.com/permissions**
Further permissions questions can be e-mailed to **permissionrequest@cengage.com**

ExamView® and *ExamView Pro*® are registered trademarks of FSCreations, Inc. Windows is a registered trademark of the Microsoft Corporation used herein under license. Macintosh and Power Macintosh are registered trademarks of Apple Computer, Inc. Used herein under license.

Library of Congress Control Number: 2007941007

ISBN-13: 978-1-4283-1895-3

ISBN-10: 1-4283-1895-X

Delmar
5 Maxwell Drive
Clifton Park, NY 12065-2919
USA

Cengage Learning products are represented in Canada by Nelson Education, Ltd.

For your lifelong learning solutions, visit **delmar.cengage.com**

Visit our corporate website at **cengage.com**

Notice to the Reader

Publisher does not warrant or guarantee any of the products described herein or perform any independent analysis in connection with any of the product information contained herein. Publisher does not assume, and expressly disclaims, any obligation to obtain and include information other than that provided to it by the manufacturer. The reader is expressly warned to consider and adopt all safety precautions that might be indicated by the activities described herein and to avoid all potential hazards. By following the instructions contained herein, the reader willingly assumes all risks in connection with such instructions. The publisher makes no representations or warranties of any kind, including but not limited to, the warranties of fitness for particular purpose or merchantability, nor are any such representations implied with respect to the material set forth herein, and the publisher takes no responsibility with respect to such material. The publisher shall not be liable for any special, consequential, or exemplary damages resulting, in whole or part, from the readers' use of, or reliance upon, this material.

Printed in the U.S.A.
2 3 4 5 10

Milady's Standard Esthetics: Fundamentals Exam Review

Foreword

Milady's Standard Esthetics: Fundamentals Exam Review has been revised to follow the type of skin care questions most frequently used by states and by the national testing, conducted under the auspices of the National-Interstate Council of State Boards of Cosmetology.

This review book is designed to be of major assistance to students in preparing for the state license examinations. The exclusive concentration on multiple-choice test items reflects the fact that all state board examinations and national testing examinations are confined to this type of question.

Questions on the state board examinations in different states will not be exactly like these and may not touch upon all the information covered in this review. But students who diligently study and practice their work as taught in the classroom and who use this book for test preparation and review should receive higher grades on both classroom and license examinations.

Part 1: Orientation

CHAPTER 1—HISTORY AND CAREER OPPORTUNITIES IN ESTHETICS

1. Skin care was practiced in early times _____.
   - a. to look appealing
   - b. to improve hunting
   - c. for self-preservation
   - d. for greater fertility _____

2. The _____ were the first to use cosmetics in an extravagant way.
   - a. Egyptians
   - b. Mayans
   - c. Neanderthals
   - d. English _____

3. Why did ancient Hebrews use cosmetics?
   - a. beautification
   - b. tribal purposes
   - c. religious ceremonies
   - d. bodily health _____

4. What were the Romans most famous for?
   - a. headdresses
   - b. clothing
   - c. baths
   - d. versatility _____

5. The ancient Asians adhered to a high standard of:
   - a. Christianity
   - b. grooming and appearance
   - c. childbearing
   - d. all answers _____

6. _____ was introduced in the twentieth century.
   - a. Botox®
   - b. Retin-A®
   - c. Alpha hydroxy acid
   - d. all answers _____

7. What do estheticians focus on?
   - a. preventive skin care
   - b. maintenance of healthy skin
   - c. makeup
   - d. all answers _____

8. Camouflage therapy involves minimizing or disguising the appearance of:
   - a. scars and fresh incisions
   - b. protruding chins
   - c. narrow eyes
   - d. all answers _____

9. Ancient people used coloring matter on which part(s) of their body?
   - a. hair
   - b. skin
   - c. nails
   - d. all answers _____

10. Women of the Middle Ages wore colored makeup on their:
    - a. cheeks and lips
    - b. eyes and eyebrows
    - c. chin and center of forehead
    - d. cheeks and chin _____

11. How did the Greeks view the human body?
   a. god
   b. gift
   c. temple
   d. accessory

   _____

12. Women of status who lived during the Age of Extravagance colored their cheeks:
   a. crimson red
   b. bright pink or orange
   c. pink only
   d. only if they were in line for the throne

   _____

13. Which services do estheticians typically perform in a spa setting?
   a. facials, waxing, body treatments, and laser hair removal
   b. facials, waxing, deep peels, and hair removal
   c. facials, waxing, body treatments, and makeup services
   d. facials, waxing, leg treatments, and makeup services

   _____

14. How do estheticians and medical a estheticians differ?
   a. no difference
   b. medical a estheticians must earn a special degree from a medical school in order to be licensed
   c. medical a estheticians provide esthetic services in a medical setting
   d. medical a estheticians must complete more school hours prior to licensing

   _____

15. Teachers, supervisors, directors, or school owners must possess_____ in order to be successful.
   a. a good sense of commercial operations
   b. a thorough knowledge of business
   c. the ability to direct and get along with people
   d. all answers

   _____

CHAPTER 2—YOUR PROFESSIONAL IMAGE

1. You can relieve stress by:
   - a. biking
   - b. swimming
   - c. running
   - d. all answers   ____

2. The method of managing your time wisely is called:
   - a. time budgeting
   - b. time management
   - c. being time wise
   - d. scheduling   ____

3. A well-developed attitude includes:
   - a. having values and goals
   - b. being naive
   - c. being set in your ways
   - d. life experience   ____

4. Professional ethics are expressed through your:
   - a. work habits
   - b. human relations skills
   - c. honesty
   - d. all answers   ____

5. Your professional image consists of your outward appearance and the conduct you exhibit in the _____.
   - a. workplace
   - b. community
   - c. classroom
   - d. employee lounge   ____

6. You can help create a stress-free and productive environment by focusing on:
   - a. team work
   - b. a partnership
   - c. a relaxed atmosphere
   - d. productivity   ____

7. Estheticians must practice within:
   - a. their license
   - b. their salon's business license
   - c. the school's certification
   - d. their treatment room   ____

8. What does personal hygiene entail?
   - a. sanitary practices
   - b. personal habits
   - c. attractive image
   - d. water temperatures   ____

9. What is true beauty rooted in?
   - a. good health
   - b. skin care products
   - c. age intervention
   - d. facial services   ____

10. Good posture includes:
    a. holding your shoulders level and relaxed
    b. looking up and elongating the neck
    c. sitting with your back rounded
    d. bending at the neck
    _____

11. Life skills can do what for your personal development?
    a. prepare you to live as a mature adult
    b. prepare you to embark on your new career
    c. help you get along better with people
    d. all answers
    _____

12. A strong work ethic includes:
    a. supporting the receptionist in the hopes of receiving more
       bookings
    b. being at work as long as your clients want you to be
    c. supporting your manager and salon owner
    d. only giving back to those who have first given to you
    _____

13. According to the guidelines for success, being kind to yourself
    means:
    a. rewarding yourself with little treats for a job well done
    b. putting a stop to self-critical and negative thoughts
    c. accepting your faults
    d. all answers
    _____

14. The two types of goals are:
    a. short-term and long-term
    c. medium and long-term
    b. immediate and future
    d. immediate and one-year
    _____

15. To ensure that you are staying on track with your goal, what
    should you do?
    a. do not set a deadline; you might fail
    b. write down your goal in explicit detail
    c. read your goal every two months
    d. reexamine your goal often
    _____

16. What does time management enable you to do?
    a. live a healthy life
    b. get everything done on your list of things to do
    c. not forget appointments
    d. all answers
    _____

4

17. Time management teaches you to:
    a. reward yourself for a job well done
    b. prioritize your tasks
    c. learn problem-solving techniques and use them
    d. all answers
    ____

18. The average facial treatment time—including additional
    consultation and retail responsibilities—generally totals:
    a. 1 hour 30 minutes   c. 1 hour 15 minutes
    b. 1 hour 45 minutes   d. 2 hours
    ____

CHAPTER 3—COMMUNICATING FOR SUCCESS

1. Besides having excellent technical skills, what must you master to succeed in the skin care business?
   a. art of communication
   b. gift of the gab
   c. in-depth medical knowledge
   d. positive thinking ____

2. An intake form is also called a(n):
   a. client history or client profile
   b. admission card or new client survey
   c. client card or portfolio
   d. client questionnaire or consultation form ____

3. Your client should always sign a(n)_____ prior to more aggressive skin care treatments.
   a. medical insurance form   c. intake form
   b. allergy history   d. consent form ____

4. When should a client consultation be done?
   a. prior to every service   c. twice yearly
   b. change of season   d. every birthday ____

5. You should cover _____ during a consultation.
   a. client's lifestyle   c. client's emotional state
   b. all key points   d. all answers ____

6. _____ is not a skin type.
   a. Normal skin   c. Oily skin
   b. Hyperpigmentation   d. Combination skin ____

7. The salon manager is generally responsible for:
   a. daily maintenance   c. quality of client services
   b. daily operations   d. all answers ____

8. When dealing with difficult people, you should always:
   a. respect boundaries
   b. think before you speak or act
   c. be assertive but respectful
   d. all answers ____

9. There is a huge difference between being right and:
   a. winning the argument   c. being correct
   b. being righteous   d. bonding with your client ____

10. Any time you have an aggressive client who is not responding to your best efforts to communicate effectively, you should:
    a. seek the aid and advice of your manager
    b. seek the aid of your most trusted coworker
    c. give the client whatever she wants to make her happy
    d. call the salon hotline ____

11. Customer service is central to:
    a. retail
    b. having a good phone system
    c. location of front desk
    d. success ____

12. You need to understand _____ before you can understand others.
    a. skin care services
    b. your family
    c. yourself
    d. your limitations ____

13. We like to interact with_____ when we feel secure.
    a. other estheticians
    b. interactive retail displays
    c. interactive Web sites
    d. other people ____

14. You should take care of _____ first.
    a. yourself
    b. your clients
    c. your friends
    d. your spouse ____

15. Communication is:
    a. e-mail, text messaging, cell phones
    b. sharing information between two people
    c. writing often
    d. successfully sharing information between two people ____

16. What should you do when you have an unhappy client on your hands?
    a. offer to redo the service as soon as you possibly can
    b. if the service cannot be redone, explain to the client exactly why this is the case
    c. ask for the assistance of your manager
    d. all answers ____

17. Every action brings about a reaction means:
    a. we cause chain reactions
    b. a quality service creates more quality services
    c. everything we do—good or bad—elicits a response from others
    d. all answers ____

18. The opposite of having a pleasant tone of voice is:
    a. rapid, jumbled speech
    b. a raspy voice
    c. feeling cranky
    d. sounding nasal
    ____

19. When dealing with a dissatisfied client, you should:
    a. argue with her
    b. try to move on to the solution
    c. debate each point
    d. not say a word
    ____

20. An employee evaluation is a formal meeting where:
    a. your progress, work habits, and skill levels are discussed
    b. new goals are set or current ones are reviewed
    c. compensation is discussed
    d. all answers
    ____

21. When giving a consultation, what should you have at your fingertips?
    a. vendor pamphlets   c. intake form
    b. before-and-after pictures d. all answers
    ____

22. Which of the following questions are not part of a 10-step consultation?
    a. skin type, skin conditions, Fitzpatrick typing
    b. lifestyle, sun exposure
    c. repeat questions
    d. marital status, children
    ____

23. In a salon/employee situation, what is the best way to handle tardy clients?
    a. follow your salon's late policy; still take the client, if you have room
    b. establish your own late policy and stick to it
    c. take them, even if you make other clients wait
    d. ask them to find another esthetician
    ____

24. What is an important step when determining why a client is unhappy?
    a. ask for specifics about the situation
    b. find out who is at fault, and start from that point
    c. check to see if she has a history of complaining
    d. check to see if she purchased products from your salon
    ____

25. When you interact with fellow staffers, you should:
    a. be honest and sensitive   c. remain objective
    b. remain neutral   d. all answers   _____

26. Gossiping with coworkers is permitted when:
    a. clients cannot hear what you are saying
    b. you trust the other person not to repeat what you are saying
    c. you are not on the salon premises
    d. it is never alright to gossip with coworkers   _____

Part 2: General Sciences

CHAPTER 4—INFECTION CONTROL: PRINCIPLES AND PRACTICE

1. What does MSDS stand for?
   a. Material Sensitivity Data Sheet
   b. Material Safety Data Sheet
   c. Material Sheet of Data Statistics
   d. Manufacturer Safety Data Sheet _____

2. _____ protect(s) clients' health, safety, and welfare.
   a. State regulatory agencies   c. State council
   b. Food and Drug Administration   d. Board of Governors _____

3. What will hospital grade and tuberculocidal disinfectants kill?
   a. bacteria   c. viruses
   b. fungi   d. all answers _____

4. The study of microbes is called:
   a. bacteriology   c. pathogenic studies
   b. microbiology   d. microscopic analysis _____

5. What are pus-forming bacteria that grow in clusters similar to grapes called?
   a. staphylococci   c. spirilla
   b. diplococci   d. streptococci _____

6. Tetanus, typhoid fever, tuberculosis, and diphtheria are caused by:
   a. staphylococci   c. diplococci
   b. bacilli   d. none of the above _____

7. _____ bacteria include treponema papillida.
   a. Streptococci   c. Bacilli
   b. Staphylococci   d. Spirilla _____

8. _____ can cause food poisoning and toxic shock syndrome.
   a. Staphylococci   c. Cocci
   b. Bacilli   d. none of the above _____

9. Communicable or _____diseases can be spread from one person to another.
   a. pathogenic   c. transferable
   b. contagious   d. non-contagious _____

10. The presence of pus indicates:
    a. infection
    b. a pimple
    c. leukemia
    d. an immune deficiency disorder _____

11. A(n)_____ sterilizes equipment by using steam under pressure.
    a. steamer
    b. autoclave
    c. full-spectrum sterilizer
    d. infusion _____

12. Isopropyl alcohol must be no less than __ % strength to disinfect tools.
    a. 99%
    b. 80%
    c. 70%
    d. 100% _____

13. Sodium hypochlorite is:
    a. rubbing alcohol
    b. witch hazel
    c. household bleach
    d. hydrogen peroxide _____

14. How do you mix disinfectant and water?
    a. pour the water into the disinfectant
    b. pour the disinfectant into the water
    c. gently shake both liquids until they emulsify
    d. the solution should stand for five minutes before stirring _____

15. What is the proper way to dispose of lancets and other sharp implements?
    a. put them in a closed trash receptacle
    b. put them in a sharps box
    c. dispose of them in a container labeled *hazardous waste*
    d. mail them back to the manufacturer _____

16. After performing a service or cleaning up contaminated implements and surfaces, what should you do with your latex gloves?
    a. turn them inside out as you take them off and put them in a biohazard trash receptacle
    b. put them in a trash bin with a closed lid
    c. turn them inside out, powder them, and reuse
    d. soak them in bleach for 10 minutes and reuse _____

17. What should you do when a client has an infection?
    a. decline the service
    b. apply a solution of quats on the sore
    c. apply a 5% solution of phenol on the wound
    d. apply rubbing alcohol to the infection _____

18. Which organisms can be spread through contact with a bloodborne pathogen?
    a. hepatitis B
    b. HIV-1
    c. hepatitis C
    d. all answers _____

19. How do anthrax and tetanus bacilli withstand long periods of famine, dryness, and unsuitable temperatures?
    a. form a waxy outer shell
    b. suspended animation
    c. adapt to the conditions
    d. burrow into other microbes _____

20. Motile bacteria:
    a. move about through dust and air
    b. independently move about
    c. are transferred within the substance in which they settle
    d. all answers _____

21. The HIV virus can be passed from one person to the next during a salon service by:
    a. entering the bloodstream through cuts and sores when using a contaminated tool
    b. airborne pathogens
    c. floating in a disinfected pedicure bowl
    d. having bloodborne pathogens in the steamer _____

22. Natural immunity is:
    a. acquired through already having had the disease, or receiving an inoculation for the disease
    b. having a healthy immune system
    c. a naturally inherited resistance to a disease
    d. all answers _____

23. Acquired immunity is the result of:
    a. having had the disease, or receiving an inoculation against the disease.
    b. acquired immunity is the same as natural immunity
    c. having inherited immunity to a disease
    d. coming in contact with an infected partner and building resistance to the pathogen over a period of time. _____

24. What can pathogenic bacteria cause?
    a. a cold
    b. infection
    c. flu
    d. viral meningitis _____

25. Formalin is a(n):
    a. safe material that is routinely used by salons to fumigate implements in a dry cabinet sanitizer
    b. unsafe material that was once routinely used by salons to fumigate implements in a dry cabinet sanitizer
    c. chemical made from alcohol
    d. non-virucidal disinfectant _____

26. What do you risk when you mix chemicals in higher concentrations than recommended by the manufacturer?
    a. solution will be too strong for salon standards
    b. solution may be less effective
    c. more effective solution
    d. spontaneous combustion _____

27. OSHA guidelines address issues relating to handling, mixing, storing, and disposing of product; general safety; and your right to know the _____ in the products you use in the workplace.
    a. benefits of the ingredients   c. hazardous ingredients
    b. promised results   d. all answers _____

28. What do non-pathogenic bacteria do?
    a. help to spread diseases
    b. break down food, protect against infection, and stimulate the immune system
    c. harm the human race
    d. cause infections _____

29. The two categories of bacteria are:
    a. pathogenic and non-pathogenic
    b. staphylococci and spirilla
    c. non-pathogenic and flagella
    d. pathogenic and cocci _____

30. Which answer best describes disinfection?
    a. using a chemical that kills most microorganisms on hard, non-porous surfaces.
    b. using a chemical that kills all microorganisms
    c. using UV light to disinfect implements
    d. using a chemical that significantly reduces the number of pathogens on a hard surface _____

31. What are dirt, oils, and microbes?
    a. pathogens   c. contaminants
    b. infectants   d. debris _____

32. What should you wear when disinfecting implements?
    a. goggles and gloves   c. safety glasses
    b. face mask   d. non-porous apron   ____

33. Cocci are transmitted:
    a. in the air, in dust, or within the substance in which they settle
    b. on top of parasites
    c. via flagella or cilia
    d. only through sexual relations   ____

34. Universal Precautions are standard infection-control practices
    that entail:
    a. treating all clients as if they were contaminated
    b. assuming all tissue (even dead skin) is hazardous
    c. treating only live skin like it has been soaked in tainted blood
    d. taking precautions when clients have contagious diseases   ____

35. A general infection is:
    a. a pus-filled lesion
    b. the result of a pathogen that is carried by the bloodstream to
       different parts of the body
    c. the result of a pathogen that enters the body through the skin
    d. indicated by pus in the bloodstream   ____

36. An aseptic procedure involves properly handling disinfected equipment:
    a. to prevent contamination before they are used on a client
    b. to prevent contamination after they are used on a client
    c. while being used on a client
    d. once the client exits the room   ____

37. Breaks in the skin, mouth, nose, eyes, or ears and unprotected
    sex are what?
    a. ways for pathogens to enter the body
    b. ways for non-pathogenic bacteria to cause infections
    c. infection points
    d. all answers   ____

38. A fourth-degree burn involves injury to:
    a. muscles, ligaments, tendons, nerves, blood vessels, and bones
    b. all layers of the skin, causing blistering, swelling, and scarring
    c. upper layers of the skin with no blisters or open skin
    d. top two layers of the skin, and shows redness and blisters   ____

CHAPTER 5—GENERAL ANATOMY AND PHYSIOLOGY

1. The basic unit of all living things is a(n):
   a. nano cell
   b. cell
   c. atom
   d. nucleus
   ____

2. What is the colorless, jelly-like substance in cells where food elements and water are present?
   a. wastes
   b. DNA
   c. nucleoplasm
   d. protoplasm
   ____

3. Anabolism is what type of metabolism?
   a. thyroid
   b. constructive
   c. destructive
   d. obstructive
   ____

4. _____ involves complex compounds being broken down into smaller ones.
   a. Canabolism
   b. Catabolism
   c. Anabolism
   d. Metabolism
   ____

5. What are bone, cartilage, ligament, tendon, fascia, and fat or adipose tissue?
   a. epithelial tissue
   b. muscular tissue
   c. connective tissue
   d. nerve tissue
   ____

6. The special cells in nerve tissue are called:
   a. neurons
   b. protons
   c. spinal cells
   d. neuropathic
   ____

7. There are ____ major systems in the human body.
   a. 9
   b. 12
   c. 11
   d. 13
   ____

8. The _____ is the foundation of the body.
   a. exoskeleton
   b. skeletal system
   c. bony network
   d. calcium deposits
   ____

9. White and red blood cells are produced by the _____ system.
   a. skeletal
   b. muscular
   c. nervous
   d. lymph vascular
   ____

10. There are _____ bones in the human body.
    a. 204
    b. 206
    c. 203
    d. 209
    ____

11. The human skull is made up of ___ bones.
    a. 20   c. 22
    b. 23   d. 27   _____

12. The _____ is not a face bone.
    a. palatine   c. mandible
    b. carpus   d. maxillary   _____

13. What do the clavicle and scapula form?
    a. hand   c. upper arm
    b. shoulder   d. hip   _____

14. Over _____ muscles are found in the human body.
    a. 600   c. 700
    b. 500   d. 350   _____

15. Muscle tissue is not stimulated by:
    a. dry ice   c. light rays
    b. moist heat   d. heat rays   _____

16. The _____ draws the corner of the mouth out and back, as in grinning.
    a. risorius   c. zygomaticus
    b. latissimus dorsi   d. mentalis   _____

17. The biceps, deltoid, and triceps enable movement in the:
    a. neck and shoulder   c. arm and hand
    b. arm and shoulder   d. fingers and wrist   _____

18. Which system is responsible for coordinating activities both inside and outside of the body?
    a. nervous   c. endocrine
    b. skeletal   d. circulatory   _____

19. _____ supply every square inch of the human body.
    a. Neurons   c. Nerves
    b. Fibers   d. Sensors   _____

20. How many cranial nerves arise from the base of the brain and the brain stem?
    a. 8   c. 13
    b. 10   d. 12   _____

21. The fifth cranial nerve is also known as the:
    a. trifacial   c. trifocal
    b. bifacial   d. bifocal   _____

18

22. The buccal nerve affects the:
    a. muscles of the mouth
    b. external ear and skin above the temple
    c. muscles of the upper part of the cheek
    d. the point and lower side of the nose _____

23. What does the infratrochlear nerve affect?
    a. skin of the forehead, scalp, eyebrow, and upper eyelid
    b. external ear and skin above the temple up to the top of the skull
    c. muscles of the upper part of the cheek
    d. membrane of the nose _____

24. The _____ is the body's pump.
    a. kidneys   c. hypothalamus
    b. brain   d. heart _____

25. There are ____ chambers and ____ valves in the human heart.
    a. four, four   c. four, three
    b. three, four   d. two, two _____

26. The largest artery in the body is the:
    a. hemoglobin   c. vein
    b. plasma   d. aorta _____

27. There are _____ pints of blood in the human body.
    a. 8–10   c. 9–10
    b. 10–12   d. 10 _____

28. The _____ helps to equalize the body's temperature and works with the immune system to protect the body from harmful microorganisms.
    a. temporalis   c. hypothalamus
    b. blood   d. none of the above _____

Endoc .

29. Which system contains glands that affect the growth, development, sexual activities, and health of the entire body?
    a. digestive   c. integumentary
    b. circulatory   d. endocrine _____

endoc.

30. What are the two main glands that make up the endocrine system?
    a. pineal and pituitary   c. hormones and pheromones
    b. exocrine and endocrine   d. adrenal and metabolic _____

31. Another name for the digestive system is:
    a. enzymatic   c. circulatory
    b. gastrointestinal   d. stomach _____

32. The primary protection for the respiratory system is (are) the:
    a. ribs   c. lungs
    b. white blood cells   d. diaphragm   _____

33. Which of the following is part of the brain?
    a. central nervous system   c. peripheral
    b. cerebrum   d. autonomic   _____

34. What do your lungs absorb into the blood when you inhale?
    a. oxygen
    b. carbon dioxide
    c. a mixture of oxygen and carbon dioxide
    d. atmospheric gases   _____

35. What gas is expelled when exhaling?
    a. carbon gases   c. carbon monoxide
    b. oxygen   d. carbon dioxide   _____

36. Tissues are made up of:
    a. layers of cells
    b. skin
    c. similar cells that perform a particular function
    d. dissimilar cells that are attracted to each other, forming a layer   _____

37. The largest, most complex nerve tissue in the human body is
    found in the:
    a. liver   c. abdomen
    b. face   d. brain   _____

38. What are neurons?
    a. building blocks of muscles
    b. primary structural units of the nervous system
    c. sources of most headaches
    d. all answers   _____

39. What carries water, oxygen, food, and secretions to all cells of
    the body?
    a. lymph   c. heart
    b. body fluids   d. blood   _____

40. Nerve tissue is responsible for:
    a. carrying messages to and from the brain
    b. helping control bodily functions
    c. helping coordinate bodily functions
    d. all answers   _____

41. The dense, active protoplasm found in the center of the cell is called:
    a. occipitalis
    c. epithelial
    b. protoplasm
    d. nucleus
    ____

42. The orbicularis oculi and corrugator are muscles of the:
    a. mouth
    c. cheeks
    b. eyebrow
    d. forehead
    ____

43. The epicranius muscle includes the occipitalis and the:
    a. frontalis
    c. triangularis
    b. levator anguli oris
    d. mentalis
    ____

44. Blood aids in protecting the body from harmful bacteria and infections through the action of:
    a. white blood cells
    c. hemoglobin
    b. red blood cells
    d. platelets
    ____

45. The skin's accessory organs include:
    a. oil glands
    c. sensory receptors
    b. sweat glands
    d. all answers
    ____

46. _____ is the dense, active protoplasm found in the center of the cell.
    a. The nucleus
    c. Deoxyribonucleic acid
    b. The core
    d. Cytoplasm
    ____

47. Dendrites are nerve fibers that receive impulses from other _____.
    a. stimuli
    c. neurons
    b. reflexes
    d. cells
    ____

48. Sensory or afferent nerves carry impulses from the sense organs to the brain, where sensations of _____ are recognized.
    a. taste, smell, and pain
    c. heat and sight
    b. touch and cold
    d. all answers
    ____

49. The _____ system is also called the circulatory system.
    a. cardiovascular
    c. heart
    b. integumentary
    d. endocrine
    ____

50. What percentage of the blood is water?
    a. 70%
    c. 65%
    b. 80%
    d. 60%
    ____

51. The _____ are the principal veins of the head, face, and neck.
    a. occipital artery and superficial temporal artery
    b. internal and external jugular veins
    c. exocrine and endocrine veins
    d. none of the above   ____

52. The ulnar and _____ arteries are primary blood supplies for the arms and hands.
    a. internal carotid   c. radial
    b. infraorbital   d. posterior auricular   ____

53. Blood to the _____ is supplied by the supraorbital artery.
    a. upper eyelid and forehead
    b. scalp, the area behind and above the ear, and the skin behind the ear
    c. muscles of the eye
    d. temples   ____

54. The infraorbital artery is responsible for supplying blood to the _____.
    a. temples
    b. side of the nose
    c. eye muscles
    d. scalp and back of the head up to the crown   ____

55. _____ involves breaking down food by mechanical and chemical means.
    a. Peristalsis   c. Absorption
    b. Digestion   d. Digestive enzymes   ____

56. What is body elimination called?
    a. peristalsis   c. catabolism
    b. defecation   d. anabolism   ____

57. How does the excretory system purify the body?
    a. excreting perspiration   c. excreting urine
    b. discharging bile   d. all answers   ____

Endocrine 58. How do fluctuating hormones adversely affect the skin?
    a. acne
    b. unwanted facial hair color and growth
    c. darker areas of pigmentation
    d. all answers   *D* ____

22

59. Define *anatomy*:
    a. study of living things
    b. study of the functions or activities performed by the body's structures
    c. study of the structures of the body that can be seen with the naked eye
    d. study of microorganisms   _____

60. What is physiology?
    a. study of the functions and activities performed by the body structures
    b. science of the structure of organisms, or of their parts, that can be seen with the naked eye
    c. study of life forms
    d. study of microorganisms   _____

61. Define *histology*:
    a. microscopic anatomy
    b. science of the structure of organisms or of their parts that can be seen with the naked eye.
    c. study of germs
    d. study of life forms   _____

62. Favorable conditions that encourage new cell reproduction and growth include:
    a. adequate supply of food   c. adequate supply of water
    b. adequate supply of oxygen   d. all answers   _____

63. Metabolism is essential to all living organisms because it:
    a. nourishes cells   c. carries away toxins
    b. purifies cells   d. all answers   _____

64. Identify the primary role of connective tissue:
    a. supports, protects, and binds together other tissues of the body
    b. provides a protective covering on body surfaces
    c. facilitates movements of joints
    d. all answers   _____

65. An organ is:
    a. a group of tissues that perform a specific function
    b. any group of tissues
    c. a group of tissues that perform non-specific functions
    d. a group of tissues that discharge bile   _____

66. Bones of the cranium include:
    a. sphenoid and ethmoid   c. parietal and occipital
    b. frontal and temporal   d. all answers   _____

67. The thorax or chest is made up of:
    a. sternum (breast bone) and spine
    b. ribs
    c. connective cartilage
    d. all answers _____

68. The bones of the arm and hand do not include the:
    a. ulna and radius
    b. ethmoid
    c. metacarpus and phalanges
    d. carpus _____

69. The muscular system:
    a. covers skeleton tissue
    b. shapes skeleton tissue
    c. supports skeleton tissue
    d. all answers _____

70. Muscle tissue includes:
    a. striated and nonstriated
    b. striated, nonstriated, and cardiac
    c. auricularis and aponeurosis
    d. levator, striated, and nonstriated _____

71. Supinators are muscles that:
    a. rotate the radius outward
    b. rotate the palm upward
    c. rotate the ulna outward
    d. create movement of the wrists _____

72. Functions of the cerebrum include:
    a. controls movement, coordinates voluntary muscular activity,
       and maintains balance and equilibrium
    b. sends messages such as thought, hearing, and sight
    c. connects the spinal cord to the brain
    d. acts as a relay station for sensory impulses and plays a role
       in the recognition of pain and temperature in the body _____

73. Efferent nerves:
    a. act as sensory-motor nerves that supply the fingers
    b. serve as the chief motor nerves of the face
    c. carry impulses from the brain to the muscles to produce
       movement
    d. serve as the chief sensory nerves of the face and as the
       motor nerves of the muscles that control chewing _____

74. Identify the chief sensory nerve of the face:
    a. fifth cranial nerve
    b. seventh cranial nerve
    c. fourth cranial nerve
    d. third cranial nerve _____

75. Branches of the fifth cranial nerve include:
    a. ophthalmic nerve
    b. mandibular nerve
    c. maxillary nerve
    d. all answers
    ____

76. The mandibular nerve affects the:
    a. skin of the forehead, scalp, eyebrow, and upper eyelid
    b. muscles of the chin and lower lip
    c. upper area of the cheek
    d. point and lower side of the nose
    ____

77. The greater auricular nerve affects the:
    a. front and sides of the neck as far down as the breastbone
    b. scalp as far up as the top of the head
    c. scalp and muscles behind the ear
    d. face, ears, neck, and parotid gland
    ____

78. The principle nerves supplying the superficial parts of the arm and hand include:
    a. digital and radial
    b. median
    c. ulnar
    d. all answers
    ____

79. The blood vascular system includes the:
    a. heart and arteries
    b. veins
    c. capillaries
    d. all answers
    ____

80. The thyroid gland:
    a. controls how quickly the body burns energy, makes protein, and how sensitive the body should be to other hormones
    b. affects the growth, development, sexual activities, and health of the entire body
    c. purifies the body
    d. performs the function of reproducing and perpetuating the human race

    Endocrine

    A
    ____

81. Identify the purpose of the pancreas:
    a. secretes enzyme-producing cells that are responsible for digesting carbohydrates, proteins, and fats
    b. releases directly into the bloodstream hormones that influence the welfare of the entire body
    c. spongy tissues composed of microscopic cells in which inhaled air is exchanged for carbon dioxide during the breathing cycle
    d. purifies the body by aiding in the elimination of waste matter

    Endocrine

    A
    ____

82. The _____ play(s) a key role in the excretory system.
    a. kidneys and liver
    c. large intestine and lungs
    b. skin
    d. all answers   _____

83. The respiratory system is composed of the:
    a. nose and lungs
    c. lungs and throat
    b. lungs and diaphragm
    d. lungs and ribs   _____

CHAPTER 6—BASICS OF CHEMISTRY

1. The human body's daily functioning is based on:
   a. reflexes
   b. perception
   c. chemical reactions
   d. all answers
   _____

2. Rusting iron and burning wood are examples of changes in:
   a. chemical properties
   b. physical properties
   c. weight
   d. shape
   _____

3. The lightest element on earth is:
   a. oxygen
   b. hydrogen
   c. water
   d. air
   _____

4. The most abundant element found on earth is:
   a. hydrogen
   b. nitrogen
   c. oxygen
   d. water
   _____

5. Four-fifths of the air in our atmosphere is made up of:
   a. oxygen
   b. hydrogen
   c. nitrogen
   d. carbon dioxide
   _____

6. _____ makes up about 65% of the human body and covers 75% of the earth's surface.
   a. Water
   b. Oxygen
   c. Hydrogen
   d. Air
   _____

7. On the pH scale, _____ is neutral.
   a. 7
   b. 0
   c. 14
   d. 6.5
   _____

8. _____ substances make up the physical mixtures of solutions, suspensions and emulsions.
   a. One or more
   b. Two to four
   c. Two or more
   d. Three or more
   _____

9. Suspensions are made of _____ of two or more substances.
   a. uniform mixtures
   b. solvents
   c. unstable mixtures
   d. blended solutions
   _____

10. _____ include skin cleansers, moisturizers, and body washes.
    a. Water-in-oil emulsions
    b. Creamy products
    c. Oil-in-water emulsions
    d. Mineral oil preparations
    _____

11. In water-in-oil emulsions, droplets of water are surrounded by surfactants with their "heads" (hydrophilic ends) pointing _____ and their "tails" (lipophilic ends) pointing ___.
    a. east, west   c. out, in
    b. in, out   d. north, south   _____

12. Solutions, suspensions, and emulsions are _____ mixtures.
    a. physical   c. redox
    b. chemical   d. solvent   _____

13. A _____ is made up of two or more atoms that are chemically joined together.
    a. chain reaction   c. chain
    b. peptide   d. molecule   _____

14. What takes place when ice melts and forms water, or when water turns into steam?
    a. chemical reaction
    b. change of state
    c. different chemical is formed
    d. all answers   _____

15. The relative degree of _____ is the potential hydrogen (pH) of a substance.
    a. acidity or alkalinity   c. reactivity
    b. chemical activity   d. stability   _____

16. Anything below 7 on the pH scale is considered:
    a. neutral   c. alkaline
    b. less effective   d. acidic   _____

17. Acid mantle:
    a. is the protective barrier of the skin
    b. is a filter that only allows beneficial organisms to reach the skin
    c. facilitates light skin peels
    d. is an acid covering   _____

18. The three states of matter are:
    a. solid, gas, and air   c. solid, liquid, and gas
    b. gas, liquid, and frozen   d. solid, liquid, and steam   _____

19. How do antioxidants prevent oxidation from occurring?
    a. kill free radicals   c. expel free radicals
    b. neutralize free radicals   d. all answers   _____

20. In skin care preparations, surfactants:
    a. wet the skin
    b. disperse oil in water
    c. emulsify oil and water
    d. all answers ____

21. A _____ is a change in the state of a substance, without the formation of a new substance.
    a. physical and chemical change
    b. new chemical
    c. physical change
    d. chemical change ____

22. Two types of chemical reactions that are important to estheticians are:
    a. acid–alkali neutralization and oxidation reduction
    b. acid oxidation and oxidation reduction
    c. acid–alkali oxidation and reduction
    d. alkali neutralization and reduction ____

23. In oil-in-water emulsions:
    a. droplets of oil are dispersed in water
    b. droplets of water are dispersed in oil
    c. droplets of oil and water are dispersed in a substance
    d. all answers ____

24. Oil-in-water is:
    a. oil added to water
    b. water added to oil
    c. a large amount of oil added to a small amount of water
    d. always a mixture of oil-in-water ____

25. An unstable mixture of two or more _____ substances united with the aid of an emulsifier is an emulsion.
    a. immiscible
    b. miscible
    c. gaseous
    d. chemical ____

26. Water-in-oil emulsions are _____ than oil-in-water emulsions.
    a. greasier
    b. more resistant
    c. heavier
    d. all answers ____

27. Identify the characteristics of solid matter:
    a. definite size (volume) and a definite shape
    b. definite size (volume), but not a definite shape
    c. does not have volume or shape
    d. definite size (volume), definite shape and length ____

28. A liquid state of matter has:
    a. definite size, but not a definite shape
    b. indefinite size and shape
    c. definite size and definite shape
    d. indefinite size and indefinite shape ____

29. Identify the physical properties of a substance:
    a. color, odor, and weight
    b. density and specific gravity
    c. melting point, boiling point, and hardness
    d. all answers   _____

30. A change in the _____ is a chemical change.
    a. physical composition of a substance
    b. chemical composition of a substance
    c. shape of a substance
    d. weight of a substance   _____

31. On a pH scale, a change of one whole number:
    a. represents a hundredfold change in pH
    b. doubles the change in pH
    c. represents a tenfold change in pH
    d. triples the change in pH   _____

32. The rapid oxidation of a substance, accompanied by the production
    of heat and light, is called:
    a. combustion   c. redox
    b. reduction   d. inflammation   _____

33. Solutions, suspensions, and emulsions are differentiated by the:
    a. size of particles and solubility of the components
    b. solubility of the components only
    c. miscibility of substances only
    d. size of particles only   _____

34. Immiscible substances are:
    a. water and oil   c. not mutually soluble
    b. miscible substances   d. mutually soluble   _____

CHAPTER 7—BASICS OF ELECTRICITY

1. The pressure of the flow of electrons through a conductor is measured by:
   a. volts
   b. pulse
   c. velocity
   d. amps
   _____

2. Sinusoidal current is used during:
   a. extractions and facial toning
   b. cleansing and facial toning
   c. scalp and facial manipulations
   d. electrolysis
   _____

3. Which of the following conditions are contraindications for electrotherapy?
   a. pacemaker
   b. epilepsy
   c. open cuts or sores
   d. all answers
   _____

4. Electricity travels:
   a. 186,000 miles per second
   b. 186,000 miles per hour
   c. 186,000 miles per nanosecond
   d. 186,000 miles per millisecond
   _____

5. UVA rays can penetrate the skin down to the:
   a. internal organs
   b. epidermis
   c. dermis
   d. all answers
   _____

6. Light therapy is another name for:
   a. wave therapy
   b. ray therapy
   c. radiation
   d. phototherapy
   _____

7. Psoriasis and acne can be treated by using:
   a. ultraviolet light
   b. white light
   c. orange light
   d. red light
   _____

8. What skin benefits have LED devices been shown to provide?
   a. helps control acne
   b. improves collagen content
   c. reduces redness
   d. all answers
   _____

9. Which answer accurately describes electricity?
    a. electricity occupies space, but it does not have physical or chemical properties
    b. electricity does not occupy space, but it does have physical properties
    c. electricity does not occupy space, but it does have chemical properties
    d. electricity does not occupy space, nor does it have physical or chemical properties   _____

10. What are sparks and lightening?
    a. effects of electricity
    b. visible electricity
    c. measured in amps
    d. white and blue forms of electricity   _____

11. Electric current:
    a. is the same as voltage
    b. is a measure of power, or the rate of energy consumption, by an electrical device when it is in operation
    c. is the flow of electrons through an electrical conductor
    d. is the unit by which electrical resistance is measured   _____

12. Primary electrical modalities used in esthetics include:
    a. galvanic
    b. faradic
    c. sinusoidal and Tesla high-frequency
    d. all answers   _____

13. The two categories of electricity include:
    a. vibrating and direct
    b. alternating and static
    c. controlled and natural
    d. direct and alternating   _____

14. Estheticians use these light rays:
    a. cosmic rays
    b. blue and red wavelengths
    c. infrared rays, ultraviolet rays, and visible light
    d. all visible wavelengths only   _____

15. The electrical path from the generating source through the conductor and back to its original source is called a(n):
    a. complete circuit   c. flow of electrons
    b. electric current   d. circuit   _____

16. What is the name for a constant, even-flowing current that travels in one direction only?
    a. sinusoidal current
    c. direct current
    b. alternating current
    d. Tesla high-frequency ____

17. A rapid and interrupted current, flowing first in one direction and then in the opposite direction, is called:
    a. alternating
    c. frictional electricity
    b. Tesla high-frequency
    d. dynamic electricity ____

18. What is the function of a circuit breaker?
    a. shuts off an electric circuit at the first indication of an overload
    b. is the same as a light switch
    c. protects against using too much electricity
    d. is a switch that has been proven to be ineffective in preventing electrical overloads ____

19. An applicator for directing the electric current from the electrotherapy machine to the client's skin is called a(n):
    a. pole
    c. rod
    b. electrode
    d. applicator tip ____

20. Which of the following exclude clients from using certain ingredients or products, or having certain treatments?
    a. indications
    c. predilections
    b. reactions
    d. contraindications ____

21. In the electromagnetic spectrum, the part that can be seen with the naked eye is (are) called:
    a. gamma waves
    c. ultraviolet rays
    b. visible light
    d. infrared waves ____

22. Which skin diseases can UVB rays cause?
    a. premature aging
    c. skin cancers
    b. solar keratoses
    d. all answers ____

23. A volt is a measurement of how much electric energy is being used in:
    a. 1 second
    c. 1 millisecond
    b. 1/10 second
    d. 1 minute ____

24. What must all electrical appliances have to operate safely?
    a. at least two electrical connections
    b. at least three electrical connections
    c. an outlet
    d. one electrical connection ____

25. All of your electrical equipment must be:
   a. salon certified   c. UL certified
   b. UL tested   d. made in the United States   _____

26. Polarity indicates the _____ or _____ pole of an electric current.
   a. negative, positive   c. dominate, lesser
   b. magnetic, non-magnetic d. all answers   _____

27. How should you disconnect your equipment?
   a. grasp the plug and pull it straight out from the outlet
   b. grasp the cord and pull it straight out from the outlet
   c. grasp the plug and the cord and pull them straight out from the outlet
   d. do not unplug professional equipment   _____

28. Besides producing chemical effects, what do ultraviolet rays do?
   a. lightly peel the skin   c. kill germs
   b. soften comedones   d. smooth the skin   _____

29. UVA rays can:
   a. penetrate the dermis   c. damage fibrils
   b. damage collagen   d. all answers   _____

30. What do broad spectrum sunscreens protect against?
   a. UVA rays only   c. UVA, UVB, and UVC rays
   b. UVA and UVB rays   d. UVB rays only   _____

31. What are the advantages of sinusoidal current over faradic current?
   a. soothes the nerves
   b. penetrates deeper into muscle tissue
   c. supplies greater stimulation
   d. all answers   _____

32. What does cataphoresis accomplish?
   a. forces acidic substances deeper into tissues
   b. forces alkaline substances into the tissues
   c. softens and emulsifies grease deposits and blackheads in the hair follicles
   d. introduces water-soluble products into the skin   _____

CHAPTER 8—BASICS OF NUTRITION

1. Which answer is another name for starches?
   a. simple carbohydrates
   b. complex carbohydrates
   c. meat
   d. all answers
   ____

2. What is the function of fiber?
   a. aids in proper digestion
   b. causes constipation
   c. suspected to cause colon cancer
   d. provides needed antibodies for the body
   ____

3. Which of the following are simple carbohydrates?
   a. many vegetables
   b. fruit and candy
   c. syrups and honey
   d. all answers
   ____

4. This macronutrient is responsible for the production of materials in the sebaceous glands:
   a. fats
   b. carbohydrates
   c. linoleic acid
   d. folic acid
   ____

5. HDLs are:
   a. high density lipoproteins
   b. low density lipoproteins
   c. the same as MDLs
   d. excess calories
   ____

6. A gram of fat contains ____ calories.
   a. 10
   b. 12
   c. 8
   d. 9
   ____

7. Vitamins B and C are water soluble vitamins that:
   a. protect the inside of the cell
   b. protect the casing around the cell
   c. nourish the cell
   d. encourage oxidation of cells
   ____

8. Vitamin C helps repair the:
   a. teeth
   b. carbon
   c. skin and tissues
   d. bones
   ____

9. What percentage of water does the body contain?
   a. 70–80%
   b. 60–80%
   c. 40–80%
   d. 50–70%
   ____

10. What do proteins contain?
    a. nearly all amino acids
    b. all amino acids
    c. some amino acids
    d. no amino acids
    ____

11. Calories:
    a. fuel the body
    b. influence skin health
    c. aid in digestion
    d. zap the body of energy ____

12. _____ is(are) related to the building of tissues and all other bodily functions.
    a. Nutrition
    b. Protein
    c. Carbohydrates
    d. The environment ____

13. _____ and _____ are the foundation of healthy skin.
    a. Vitamins, moisturizer
    b. Moisturizers, skin serums
    c. Diet, water
    d. all answers ____

14. Which of the following substances is necessary for the growth and development of the human body?
    a. macronutrients
    b. lipids
    c. ceramides
    d. keratin ____

15. Which of the following are macronutrients?
    a. proteins
    b. carbohydrates
    c. fats
    d. all answers ____

16. Chains of _____ are used by every cell of the body.
    a. amino acid molecules
    b. protein molecules
    c. cells
    d. all answers ____

17. Chains of amino acid molecules are used by every cell of the body to make:
    a. skin
    b. phospholipids
    c. other proteins
    d. keratin only ____

18. Between the fibers of the dermis, there is a water-binding substance called:
    a. glycosaminoglycan
    b. hyaluronidase
    c. water-loving enzyme
    d. peroxidase ____

19. _____ include grains and certain legumes.
    a. Low fiber foods
    b. High fiber foods
    c. Complete proteins
    d. Proteins ____

20. Fats should be no more than ___ of your diet.
    a. 20%
    b. 25%
    c. 28%
    d. 30% ____

21. Retinol and _____ are different names for the same micronutrient.
    a. vitamin A
    b. vitamin B
    c. vitamin C
    d. ascorbic acid ____

22. Vitamin D is called the sunshine vitamin because:
    a. the only source of vitamin D is through exposure to sunlight
    b. UV rays optimize the synthesis of vitamin D
    c. UV rays are a source of vitamin D
    d. the skin metabolizes vitamin D from all adipose tissues when exposed to sunlight   ____

23. Vitamins, or micronutrients, _____.
    a. have no nutritional value
    b. are high in nutritional value
    c. have a moderate amount of nutritional value
    d. are the primary source of nutrition   ____

24. How many calories are in micronutrients?
    a. 10 calories per gram
    b. 100 calories per gram
    c. no calories
    d. micronutrient calories vary according to the food source   ____

25. Identify the benefit(s) of vitamin A:
    a. is an antioxidant   c. improves skin thickness
    b. improves the skin's elasticity d. all answers   ____

26. Which of the following is (are) true about vitamin A?
    a. treats acne
    b. improves the depth of wrinkles
    c. has antioxidant properties that benefit the entire body
    d. all answers   ____

27. Pyridoxine:
    a. metabolizes proteins
    b. rids the body of harmful cholesterol
    c. helps in weight management
    d. all answers   ____

28. Vitamin D deficiency causes:
    a. heart disease   c. scurvy
    b. lupus   d. rickets   ____

29. _____ include(s) niacin, riboflavin, thiamine, and pyridoxine.
    a. B vitamins   c. Vitamin C
    b. Vitamin A   d. Vitamin E   ____

30. Pantothenic acid plays a role in the:
    a. skin's barrier function   c. activity of the dermis
    b. production of keratin   d. metabolic rate   ____

31. Which of the following is a benefit of vitamin C?
    a. prevents rickets
    b. known as the sunshine vitamin
    c. FDA recommends that healthy people ingest a minimum of 1000 mgs of vitamin C a day
    d. an antioxidant that neutralizes free radical activity ____

32. Which of the following most accurately describes the role of sodium in the body?
    a. transports materials through the cell membranes and regulates water levels
    b. causes nerve and muscle irritability
    c. higher amounts may lower blood pressure
    d. all answers ____

33. _____ is aided by iron.
    a. Oxidation in the body
    b. Cholesterol and free radical production
    c. Hemoglobin and red blood cell production
    d. Hemoglobin production and oxygenation ____

34. Zinc is a trace mineral that:
    a. is important for protein synthesis
    b. promotes wound healing
    c. is important for collagen formation
    d. all answers ____

35. Each person's nutritional needs depend on:
    a. age and sex
    b. weight and physical activity
    c. body type
    d. all answers ____

36. Manganese supports:
    a. elastin formation
    c. protein and fat metabolism
    b. collagen formation
    d. stable blood sugar levels ____

37. What is the USDA food pyramid?
    a. a daily nutritional guideline
    b. the daily amount of food that individuals should consume
    c. guide for weight management
    d. chart for caloric intake ____

38. Select the correct definition for *complementary foods*:
    a. combination of two incomplete proteins that make a complete protein
    b. combination of two complete proteins that make a highly nutritious meal
    c. combination of two incompatible proteins that should never be combined
    d. combination of two incompatible proteins that create a highly nutritious meal
    _____

39. Carbohydrates:
    a. neutralize chemical sugars
    b. build up basic chemical sugars that supply energy for the body
    c. prevent the absorption of chemical sugars
    d. break down basic chemical sugars that supply energy for the body
    _____

40. Bad cholesterol in the blood is called:
    a. HDL (high-density lipoproteins)
    b. LDL (low-density lipoproteins)
    c. ALS (average lipoproteins)
    d. MDL (moderate-density lipoproteins)
    _____

41. Enzymes are:
    a. biological catalysts
    b. sugars
    c. platelets
    d. the prime substance in protoplasm
    _____

42. Fat-soluble vitamins include:
    a. vitamin E
    b. vitamin A
    c. vitamins D and K
    d. all answers
    _____

43. Vitamin K benefits include:
    a. helps strengthen capillary walls
    b. is used in some skin care preparations to help minimize dark undereye circles
    c. essential for the synthesis of proteins that are necessary for blood coagulation
    d. all answers
    _____

44. Riboflavin:
    a. works with proteins to produce energy in cells
    b. is used by cells to manufacture various amino acids and fatty acids
    c. is the major factor of skin health
    d. is used by cells to break down various amino acids and fatty acids   _____

45. To determine the amount of water you should drink each day: Take your body weight and divide by _____. Divide this number by 8.
    a. 4   c. 8
    b. 6   d. 2   _____

Part 3: Skin Sciences

CHAPTER 9—PHYSIOLOGY AND HISTOLOGY OF THE SKIN

1. The largest organ of the body is:
   - a. skin
   - b. liver
   - c. heart
   - d. endocrine glands
   _____

2. The barrier function of the skin includes:
   - a. hair
   - b. follicles
   - c. pores
   - d. acid mantle
   _____

3. Which of the following answers defines *hydro*?
   - a. oil
   - b. water
   - c. sweat
   - d. all answers
   _____

4. Identify the two layers or sections of the skin.
   - a. epidermis and dermis
   - b. epidermis and melanocytes
   - c. dermis and keratinocytes
   - d. dermis and lipids
   _____

5. Approximately what percentage of water is found in healthy skin?
   - a. 60–70%
   - b. 80%
   - c. 50–70%
   - d. 50–60%
   _____

6. Keratin and intercellular lipids are formed in the:
   - a. stratum corneum
   - b. stratum spinosum
   - c. dermis
   - d. stratum granulosum
   _____

7. Which layer of the skin produces melanin?
   - a. stratum granulosum
   - b. stratum spinosum
   - c. stratum germinativum
   - d. dermis
   _____

8. The junction where the dermis connects to the epidermis is called:
   - a. epidermis–dermis junction
   - b. epidermal–dermal junction
   - c. papilla–dermal junction
   - d. papillary–dermal junction
   _____

9. _____ aid in the production of collagen and elastin.
   - a. Adipose tissues
   - b. Glycosaminoglycans
   - c. Melanocytes
   - d. Fibroblasts
   _____

10. Subcutis or _____ tissue is found below the reticular layer.
    - a. cutaneous
    - b. collagen
    - c. basal cells
    - d. adipose
    _____

11. Identify the slender outgrowth of the scalp.
    a. hair
    b. nails
    c. eyelashes
    d. all answers

    _____

12. Which fibers stimulate the arrector pili muscles?
    a. secretory nerves
    b. follicles
    c. motor nerves
    d. goose bumps

    _____

13. Which cells in the basal layer produce pigment granules?
    a. lancets
    b. melanocytes
    c. eccrine gland cells
    d. apocrine gland cells

    _____

14. The _____ glands excrete sweat.
    a. sudoriferous
    b. hyaluronic
    c. arrector pili
    d. oil

    _____

15. What do cells need in order to survive?
    a. nourishment
    b. to proliferate
    c. protection
    d. all answers

    _____

16. What are phospholipids, glycolipids, cholesterol, triglycerides, squalene, and waxes?
    a. lipids
    b. proteins
    c. fatty acids
    d. ceramides

    _____

17. _____ of cells are replaced by the body on a daily basis.
    a. Thousands
    b. Millions
    c. Billions
    d. Trillions

    _____

18. Which of the following answers stimulates cell turnover?
    a. alpha hydroxy acids
    b. ceramides
    c. hyaluronic acid
    d. beneficial UVA rays

    _____

19. Atoms or molecules with unpaired electrons are called:
    a. oxidation
    b. UVB rays
    c. trapped radicals
    d. free radicals

    _____

20. Free radical activity causes:
    a. luminosity
    b. inflammation
    c. pimples
    d. skin cancer

    _____

21. Natural antioxidants are found in the skin.
    a. true
    b. false
    c. depends
    d. usually

    _____

22. Which of the following causes premature aging of the skin?
    a. smoking   c. certain drugs
    b. tanning   (d.) all answers   _____

23. Identify the greatest aging effect on skin:
    a. UV rays   c. some drugs
    b. alcohol   d. lack of sleep   _____

24. _____ are called the burning rays.
    a. UVA rays   c. UVB rays
    b. UVC rays   d. Infrared rays   _____

25. In order to block UVA and UVB rays, sunscreens must be:
    a. broad spectrum   c. full coverage
    b. full spectrum   d. opaque   _____

26. Estrogen protects the skin by:
    a. being anti-inflammatory   c. having antioxidant qualities
    b. repairing skin tissue   d. all answers   _____

27. An esthetician's primary role is to _____, and nourish
    the skin.
    a. preserve, protect
    b. smooth, tighten
    c. reverse aging, clear complexions
    d. prevent, prelighten   _____

28. What is the average square footage and weight of an adult's skin?
    a. 22 sq. ft.; 8–10 lbs   c. 31 sq. ft.; 15–18 lbs
    b. 10 sq. ft.; 4–5 lbs   d. 21 sq. ft.; 7–9 lbs   _____

29. What does TEWL stand for?
    (a.) transepidermal water loss   c. transepidermal lipids
    b. transitional water loss   d. transferable water lipids   _____

30. The most amazing feature of the skin is its ability to:
    a. form scars   c. heal itself
    b. stay warm   d. tan   _____

31. Which glands excrete perspiration and detoxify the body?
    a. papilla   c. sudoriferous
    b. sebaceous   d. arrector pili   _____

32. Skin absorbs:
    a. carbon dioxide   c. dirt
    b. oxygen   d. carbon monoxide   _____

33. Physiology is most accurately described as:
    a. study of the internal workings of microorganisms
    b. study of the internal workings of living organisms
    c. study of the internal workings of hair, skin, and nails
    d. study of the internal workings of genetics   ____

34. Appendages include:
    a. hair   c. sweat and oil glands
    b. nails   d. all answers   ____

35. Primary functions of the skin include:
    a. protection and sensation   c. absorption and excretion
    b. heat regulation and secretion d. all answers   ____

36. What does the skin protect against?
    a. inside elements and macroorganisms
    b. outside elements and microorganisms
    c. outside elements and macroorganisms
    d. inside elements and microorganisms   ____

37. Fat insulation keeps the body:
    a. an even temperature   c. warm
    b. warm and cool   d. operating efficiently   ____

38. The sebaceous glands:
    a. soften the skin
    b. excrete sebum
    c. protect the skin from outside elements
    d. all answers   ____

39. Identify the answer that is not a layer of the skin:
    a. stratum lucidum   c. stratum granulosum
    b. stratum germinativum   d. epithelial layer   ____

40. Lipids:
    a. protect cells from dehydration
    b. protect cells from UV rays
    c. protect cells from free radicals
    d. protect cells from white blood cells   ____

41. It is important to understand the function of each layer of the
    skin because it helps you to:
    a. correctly choose products and treatments
    b. correctly choose the delivery system
    c. correctly choose the right makeup
    d. assess a person's overall health   ____

42. Mitosis occurs in which layer of the skin?
    a. stratum germinativum   c. stratum lucidum
    b. stratum granulosum   d. stratum spinosum   ____

43. The two layers of the dermis are the:
    a. reticular and stratum spinosum
    b. reticular and stratum germinativum
    c. papillary and adipose tissue
    d. papillary and reticular   ____

44. Papillae are located:
    a. at the bottom of the follicles   c. next to the hair follicles
    b. inside the oil glands   d. inside arrector pili   ____

45. Elastin:
    a. forms elastic tissue   c. creates firmness in skin
    b. protects the dermis   d. makes the skin rigid   ____

46. Absorption of water and oxygen are:
    a. harmful to the skin
    b. dependent on UV rays
    c. the job of the dermis
    d. necessary for the skin's health   ____

47. The _____ is also referred to as the spiny layer.
    a. stratum corneum   c. stratum spinosum
    b. stratum granulosum   d. stratum lucidum   ____

48. Which answer most accurately describes the stratum corneum?
    a. translucent layer that allows sunlight to pass through the skin
    b. opaque layer that prevents sunlight from passing through
       the skin
    c. is living tissue
    d. repels free radicals   ____

49. The _____ is also called the basal layer of the epidermis.
    a. stratum corneum   c. stratum lucidum
    b. stratum granulosum   d. stratum germinativum   ____

50. The thickest layer of the skin is called the:
    a. dermis   c. stratum corneum
    b. epidermis   d. stratum spinosum   ____

51. Which answer is the proper name for cell division?
    a. division   c. genesis
    b. separation   d. mitosis   ____

CHAPTER 10—DISORDERS AND DISEASES OF THE SKIN

1. What do you call physicians who treat skin disorders and diseases?
   a. physiology experts
   b. dermatology specialists
   c. anatomy specialists
   d. dermatologists
   ____

2. Diagnosing skin conditions is not within the scope of your:
   a. jurisdiction
   b. license
   c. certification
   d. accreditation
   ____

3. When skin is injured, it can cause:
   a. tubercles
   b. tumors
   c. lesions
   d. pustules
   ____

4. Lesions that are in the early stages of development are:
   a. primary lesions
   b. secondary lesions
   c. advanced lesions
   d. flat lesions
   ____

5. The medical term for freckles is:
   a. vesicles
   b. melasma
   c. macules
   d. nodules
   ____

6. What is the correct term for an insect bite, skin allergy reaction, or sting that becomes itchy and swollen?
   a. wheal
   b. blister
   c. pustule
   d. rash
   ____

7. Scratching or scraping the skin can produce a(n):
   a. excoriation
   b. fissure
   c. keloid
   d. ulcer
   ____

8. A thin plate of epidermal cells is called:
   a. dry skin
   b. dandruff
   c. asteatosis
   d. scale
   ____

9. What is the medical term for chronic inflammation of the sebaceous glands?
   a. asteatosis
   b. acne
   c. acne excorie
   d. seborrhea
   ____

10. Inflammation, dry or oily scaling or crusting, and/or itchiness is caused by:
    a. a furuncle
    b. acne
    c. sebaceous dermatitis
    d. seborrheic dermatitis
    ____

11. Pearl-like masses of white material under the skin with no visible openings are called:
    a. boils   c. milia
    b. comedones   d. pimples   _____

12. When oilier areas of the face develop benign lesions, it is called:
    a. sebaceous hyperplasia   c. seborrhea
    b. milia   d. steatoma   _____

13. Disorders of the sudoriferous glands include:
    a. anhidrosis   c. hyperhidrosis
    b. bromhidrosis   d. all answers   _____

14. A condition characterized by bacteria and yeast that causes a foul odor is called:
    a. anhidrosis   c. bromhidrosis
    b. hyperhidrosis   d. miliaria rubra   _____

15. Perspiration deficiency caused by failure of the sweat glands is called:
    a. hyperhidrosis   c. bromhidrosis
    b. miliaria rubra   d. anhidrosis   _____

16. When excessive heat exposure causes an acute inflammatory disorder of the sweat glands, it is called:
    a. miliaria rubra   c. sebaceous hyperplasia
    b. hyperhidrosis   d. furuncle   _____

17. Atopic dermatitis is:
    a. a rash   c. eczema
    b. rosacea   d. psoriasis   _____

18. A condition characterized by painful itching and inflammation with dry or moist lesions is called:
    a. edema   c. dermatitis
    b. eczema   d. atopic dermatitis _____

19. The medical term for hives is:
    a. folliculitis   c. urticaria
    b. erythema   d. perioral dermatitis _____

20. Pruritis is a condition characterized by:
    a. scratching   c. hives
    b. rubbing   d. itching   _____

21. Spicy foods, alcohol, caffeine, exposure to extreme temperatures, heat, sun, and stress aggravate:
    a. rosacea
    b. contact dermatitis
    c. edema
    d. all answers
    _____

22. Red patches covered with white–silver scales on the scalp, elbows, knees, chest, and lower back are characteristics of:
    a. rosacea
    b. urticaria
    c. psoriasis
    d. erythema
    _____

23. The medical term for a distended capillary is:
    a. couperose skin
    b. telangiectasia
    c. folliculitis
    d. rosacea
    _____

24. Estheticians commonly develop skin allergies on the:
    a. cheeks
    b. fingers and palms
    c. backs of hands
    d. all answers
    _____

25. What can exposure to an allergen cause?
    a. allergic reaction
    b. toxic allergy
    c. anaphylactic shock
    d. hypersensitivity
    _____

26. Allergic reactions to esthetic treatments are commonly found in these areas:
    a. scalp, hair, forehead, and neckline
    b. scalp, hairline, forehead, and neckline
    c. scalp, hairline, forehead, and neck
    d. wrists, hairline, forehead, and neckline
    _____

27. Substances that can irritate the skin are:
    a. caustic
    b. oily
    c. gelatinous
    d. mineral
    _____

28. What is a port wine stain?
    a. mole
    b. melasma
    c. lentigene
    d. vascular nevus
    _____

29. The general term for dark blotchy spots on the skin is:
    a. hyperpigmentation
    b. melanin
    c. stain
    d. nevus
    _____

30. When the entire body lacks melanin, it is called:
    a. vitiligo
    b. hyperpigmentation
    c. albinism
    d. leukoderma
    _____

31. Congenital spotty hypopigmentation is called:
    a. albinism   c. vitiligo
    b. hypertrophy   d. leukoderma   _____

32. Which of the following answers is the medical term for a callus?
    a. actinic keratoses   c. keratoma
    b. keratosis pilaris   d. atrophy   _____

33. Keratosis pilaris can be treated by an esthetician with a(n)
    _____ service.
    a. manicure   c. seaweed wrap
    b. pedicure   d. exfoliation   _____

34. A thickening of the skin caused by a mass of keratinized cells is
    called:
    a. actinic keratosis   c. keratosis pilaris
    b. hyperkeratosis   d. verruca   _____

35. A non-viral flap of skin is called a:
    a. skin tag   c. port wine stain
    b. mole   d. wart   _____

36. What causes 90% of skin cancers?
    a. sun exposure   c. cosmetics
    b. chemical exposure   d. melanoma   _____

37. Photoaging can be seen in the:
    a. 30s or before   c. 20s or before
    b. 40s or before   d. teens or before   _____

38. Tanning is safe:
    a. in moderation
    b. only in the summer
    c. during the early morning hours
    d. never   _____

39. Eighty percent of sun damage occurs by age:
    a. 40   c. 20
    b. 30   d. 18   _____

40. What is the most deadly form of skin cancer?
    a. malignant melanoma
    b. squamous cell carcinoma
    c. basal cell carcinoma
    d. squamous–basal carcinoma   _____

41. Which of the following answers describes the appearance of malignant melanoma?
   a. asymmetrical
   b. uneven borders
   c. uneven color
   d. all answers
   _____

42. This term is interchangeable with *infectious* or *communicable*:
   a. bacterial conjunctivitis
   b. herpes virus
   c. communicable disease
   d. herpes zoster
   _____

43. The medical term for cold sores or fever blisters is:
   a. bacterial conjunctivitis
   b. herpes simplex virus
   c. tinea versicolor
   d. tinea
   _____

44. What is the medical term for ringworm?
   a. tinea corporis
   b. tinea versicolor
   c. verruca
   d. impetigo
   _____

45. Comedones and blemishes are symptoms of what condition?
   a. acne
   b. retention hyperkeratosis
   c. sebaceous filaments
   d. philosebaceous duct
   _____

46. P. acnes bacteria are _____, meaning they cannot live in the presence of oxygen.
   a. androgens
   b. estrogens
   c. anaerobic
   d. moist
   _____

47. Nodules with deep pockets of infection are called:
   a. pimples
   b. comedones
   c. blackheads
   d. cysts
   _____

48. Acne in the dermis that causes depressed and raised scars is called:
   a. acne
   b. bacterial acne
   c. cystic acne
   d. P. acnes
   _____

49. Acne is caused by:
   a. genetics/heredity
   b. clogged pores
   c. bacteria
   d. all answers
   _____

50. All male hormones are called:
   a. androgens
   b. estrogens
   c. testosterone
   d. sebaceous filaments
   _____

51. Which group of people is most likely to have adult acne?
   a. men
   b. women
   c. retirees
   d. Midwesterners
   _____

52. When the chin develops acne, it can be caused by:
    a. hormones   c. climate changes
    b. diet   d. pregnancy   ____

53. Which type of product causes clogged pores?
    a. comedogenic   c. water
    b. non comedogenic   d. mineral makeup   ____

54. Identify the acne irritants:
    a. MSG and minerals obtained from an ocean source
    b. iodides and fast food
    c. kelp and cheese
    d. all answers   ____

55. Grade I acne symptoms include:
    a. minor breakouts, mostly open comedones, and a few papules
    b. many closed comedones, more open comedones, and
       occasional papules and pustules
    c. red and inflamed skin and many papules and pustules
    d. cystic acne   ____

56. Red and inflamed skin, many comedones, and papules and
    pustules are characteristics of which grade of acne?
    a. Grade I   c. Grade III
    b. Grade II   d. Grade IV   ____

57. Medications that treat acne include:
    a. tretinoin (Retin-A®)   c. azelaic acid
    b. adapalene   d. all answers   ____

CHAPTER 11—SKIN ANALYSIS

1. A _____ type is something a person is born with.
    a. skin
    b. face
    c. personality
    d. all answers
    _____

2. The five different skin types are:
    a. dry, normal, combination, oily, and sensitive
    b. dry, normal, combination, oily, and acneic
    c. dehydrated, normal, combination, oily, and sensitive
    d. dehydrated, normal, combination, rough, and oily
    _____

3. Only one skin type can also be a skin condition. What is it?
    a. combination
    b. oily
    c. sensitive
    d. normal
    _____

4. When skin lacks_____, it is classified as a dry skin type.
    a. water
    b. oil
    c. reaction
    d. alipidic
    _____

5. Small follicles indicate that the skin is _____.
    a. sensitive
    b. oily
    c. dry
    d. normal
    _____

6. This skin type has an unhealthy acid mantle and skin barrier function:
    a. oily
    b. sensitive
    c. normal
    d. dry
    _____

7. Occlusive products do what?
    a. reduce transepidermal water loss
    b. encourage transepidermal water loss
    c. clog the pores
    d. combat oiliness
    _____

8. Which skin type(s) can be dehydrated?
    a. dry
    b. oily
    c. combination
    d. all answers
    _____

9. Skin that is dehydrated lacks:
    a. water
    b. oil
    c. stratum corneum
    d. cell renewal
    _____

10. When follicles go from smaller to medium just on the edge of the T-zone by the nose, the skin type is:
    a. oily
    b. dry
    c. sensitive
    d. normal
    _____

11. Blemishes develop in oily skin because the pores get clogged with:
    a. oil and dead skin cells
    b. P. acnes
    c. smog
    d. dead skin cells only ____

12. Having a good water-and-oil balance is characteristic of which skin type(s)?
    a. combination
    b. sensitive
    c. normal
    d. all answers ____

13. Products and exposure to heat or sun can easily irritate this skin type:
    a. aging
    b. fair
    c. darkly pigmented skin
    d. sensitive ____

14. The _____ is a skin typing system that shows the skin's ability to withstand sun exposure.
    a. Fitzpatrick Scale
    b. MacDonald Scale
    c. Sun Exposure Table
    d. burn factor ____

15. The Fitzpatrick Scale classifies people with very fair skin, blond or red hair, and light-colored eyes as:
    a. Type IV
    b. Type VI
    c. Type II
    d. Type I ____

16. _____ on the Fitzpatrick Scale includes Mideastern skin that tans and is rarely sensitive to the sun.
    a. Type III
    b. Type IV
    c. Type V
    d. Type VI ____

17. Different amounts of _____ are found in black, Hispanic, Asian, and Native American skin types.
    a. melanosomes
    b. hormones
    c. melanin
    d. keratinocytes ____

18. Hyperkeratosis can be defined as:
    a. excessive dead skin cell buildup and cell turnover
    b. inadequate dead cell buildup
    c. hyperpigmentation
    d. oily, thick skin ____

19. Darker skin types can suffer from _____ due to trauma, extractions, sun damage, or exfoliation.
    a. pre-inflammatory hypopigmentation
    b. post-inflammatory hyperpigmentation
    c. pre-inflammatory hyperpigmentation
    d. all answers ____

20. Which ethnic skin type is considered to be most sensitive to peels?
    a. Mediterranean   c. Asian
    b. Mideastern   d. Hispanic   _____

21. You should be most concerned about the _____ when treating skin.
    a. skin condition   c. Fitzpatrick Scale
    b. skin type   d. ethnic vs. Caucasian skin   _____

22. A person's skin condition can be influenced by:
    a. external factors only
    b. internal factors only
    c. internal and external factors
    d. all answers   _____

23. Which of the following are skin conditions?
    a. couperose, sensitive, and wrinkling
    b. dry, oily, or normal
    c. natural pigmentation
    d. all answers   _____

24. Rough areas that are caused by sun exposure and are sometimes accompanied by a layered scale or scab are characteristics of this skin condition:
    a. telangiectasias   c. adult acne
    b. hyperpigmentation   d. actinic keratosis   _____

25. Inflammatory redness is called:
    a. couperose   c. a rash
    b. erythema   d. alipidic skin   _____

26. Choose the description that best describes comedones:
    a. blackheads and whiteheads   c. blackheads only
    b. whiteheads only   d. cysts   _____

27. A blackhead can be most accurately described as a(n):
    a. closed comedone   c. open comedone
    b. pore congestion   d. blemish   _____

28. What type of skin condition is caused by smoking?
    a. acne   c. dehydrated
    b. sensitive   d. asphyxiated   _____

29. When skin is asphyxiated, what does it lack?
    a. water   c. hydrogen
    b. oxygen   d. oil   _____

30. Large blackheads around the eyes are specifically called:
    a. actinic keratosis   c. comedones
    b. lunar comedones   d. solar comedones   _____

31. When papules become infected and contain fluid, they
    are called:
    a. pustules   c. solar comedones
    b. sebaceous hyperplasia   d. keratoses   _____

32. Externally, the skin is most damaged by:
    a. smoking   c. sun exposure
    b. poor vitamin intake   d. dehydration   _____

33. What does MED stand for?
    a. midway erythemal dose
    b. minimal erythemal dose
    c. measured erythemal dose
    d. maximum erythemal dose   _____

34. MED measures:
    a. how long it takes to become red from sun exposure
    b. how long it takes to become red from environmental chemical
       exposure
    c. how long it takes to become red from chemical irritants
    d. all answers   _____

35. Skin can suffer from _____ as a result of being exposed
    to UVA rays.
    a. photoaging   c. skin cancer
    b. DNA damage   d. all answers   _____

36. UVB rays are characterized by:
    a. shorter, stronger wavelengths
    b. stronger wavelengths, but less energy
    c. going deeper into the skin than UVA rays
    d. having no ability to cause sunburn   _____

37. What are the causes of erythema?
    a. cell damage and blood vessel dilation in the basal layer
    b. cell damage and blood vessel dilation in the epidermis
    c. cell damage and blood vessel dilation in the epithelial tissue
    d. cell damage and blood vessel dilation in the dermis   _____

38. This layer of the atmosphere is responsible for absorbing UVC rays:
    a. ozone layer   c. outer space
    b. gaseous   d. cloud cover   _____

56

39. High amounts of antioxidants can be found in these foods:
    a. berries and citrus fruits
    b. citrus fruits and bananas
    c. berries and sweet potatoes
    d. all answers _____

40. A family of antioxidants known as polyphenols can be found in:
    a. green tea
    b. red grapes
    c. strawberries and pomegranates
    d. all answers _____

41. _____ for esthetic services include(s) contagious diseases.
    a. Indications   c. Contraindications
    b. The need   d. all answers _____

42. Lupus is one example of a(n) _____ disease.
    a. immune system   c. respiratory
    b. autoimmune system   d. vascular _____

43. Harsh exfoliating or waxing treatments should always be avoided when clients are taking:
    a. vitamins   c. oral steroids
    b. minerals   d. heart medications _____

44. These treatments may trigger an epileptic seizure:
    a. light or electrical treatments   c. massage
    b. body wraps   d. extractions _____

45. Clients with _____ should not receive electrical treatments.
    a. conditions warranting blood thinning medications
    b. skin allergies
    c. diabetes or vitamin deficiencies
    d. heart abnormalities or have a pacemaker _____

46. You must ask important questions, such as, "What are your skin concerns?" when:
    a. doing a consultation
    b. doing an examination of the skin
    c. filling out a skin analysis chart
    d. filling out a release form _____

47. Asking your client how their skin feels during different parts of the day provides valuable information about what?
    a. oiliness or dryness   c. combination skin
    b. dryness only   d. mature skin _____

48. Touching the skin with your fingers during a skin analysis helps you to determine whether or not the skin is:
    a. oily
    b. dry
    c. rough
    d. dehydrated ____

49. The four components of every skin analysis include?
    a. look
    b. feel
    c. ask and listen
    d. all answers ____

CHAPTER 12—SKIN CARE PRODUCTS: CHEMISTRY, INGREDIENTS, AND SELECTION

1. What is your most important tool?
   - a. product
   - b. Woods Lamp
   - c. facial machine
   - d. all answers
   _____

2. The quality of the skin can be _____ improved with professional skin care products.
   - a. slightly
   - b. somewhat
   - c. significantly
   - d. moderately
   _____

3. Skin care ingredients can be studied at a _____ level.
   - a. scientific
   - b. macroscopic
   - c. visible
   - d. molecular
   _____

4. How many different products must you know about to effectively practice professional skin care?
   - a. only the products you use
   - b. a broad spectrum of products
   - c. all popular retail products
   - d. every product on the market
   _____

5. Cosmetics are distinguished from drugs by this act:
   - a. Cosmetic Act of 1938
   - b. FDA
   - c. Cosmetics Board
   - d. drug enforcement
   _____

6. According to the Cosmetic Act of 1938, products that are made to affect the structures and/or functions of the human body are:
   - a. water
   - b. cosmetics
   - c. drugs
   - d. all answers
   _____

7. What category of ingredients cause the actual changes in the appearance of the skin?
   - a. performance
   - b. functional
   - c. cosmeceuticals
   - d. whole plant
   _____

8. Ingredients that are hypoallergenic are _____ to cause allergic reactions.
   - a. not likely
   - b. more likely
   - c. absolutely unable
   - d. definitely unable
   _____

9. Products that avoid clogging pores or causing comedones are called:
   - a. oil free
   - b. comedogenic
   - c. anhydrous
   - d. non comedogenic
   _____

10. Anhydrous products include:
    a. lip balms   c. oil serums
    b. petrolatum-based products   d. all answers   _____

11. Substances used to lubricate and moisturize the skin are called:
    a. lotions   c. emollients
    b. preservatives   d. carbomers   _____

12. Substances that coat the skin and reduce friction belong to this category:
    a. lubricants   c. oils
    b. emollients   d. mineral oil   _____

13. Ingredients that are beneficial to dry skin are:
    a. fatty acids   c. rubbing alcohol
    b. sebum   d. fatty materials   _____

14. _____ include oleic acid, steric acid, and caprylic acid.
    a. Fatty alcohols   c. Silicones
    b. Fatty esters   d. Fatty acids   _____

15. Surfactants:
    a. improve moisture   c. improve spreadability
    b. protect the skin   d. all answers   _____

16. _____ reduce the surface tension of dirt and oils on the skin's surface and form an emulsion to lift them from the skin.
    a. Detergents   c. Fresheners
    b. Emulsifiers   d. Carbomers   _____

17. Substances that are mixable with water are called:
    a. water insoluble   c. oil insoluble
    b. oily water   d. water soluble   _____

18. A treatment where aromatherapy oils are inhaled for their therapeutic benefits is called:
    a. plant oil therapy c. aromatherapy
    b. olfactory oil therapy   d. plant power   _____

19. Products that enhance the effectiveness of a preservative are called:
    a. fatty esters   c. anticontaminants
    b. fatty alcohols   d. chelating agents   _____

20. Which of the following substances adds color to cosmetics and are certified by the FDA?
    a. certified colors   c. lakes
    b. color agents   d. non-certified colors _____

21. Substances used to adjust the pH of products are called:
    a. pH balancers   c. solvents
    b. pH levelers   d. pH adjustors   _____

22. A solvent is a:
    a. humectant
    b. hydrator
    c. healing agent
    d. substance that dissolves other substances   _____

23. Plant-based ingredients are:
    a. solvents   c. botanicals
    b. humectants   d. healing agents   _____

24. Which of the following are used as natural exfoliators?
    a. jojoba beads   c. various seeds
    b. ground nuts   d. all answers   _____

25. Which acids have beneficial chemical effects on the skin?
    a. AHAs and BHAs   c. BHAs and DHAs
    b. AHAs and CHAs   d. BHAs and EHAs   _____

26. Identify the hydroxy acids:
    a. glycolic and lactic   c. malic and tartaric
    b. citric and salicylic d. all answers   _____

27. Which acids exfoliate by loosening the bonds between cells in the surface of the corneum?
    a. citric and salicylic acids   c. glycolic and lactic
    b. malic and tartaric acids   d. all answers   _____

28. Which ingredients dissolve keratin proteins on the surface of the skin?
    a. enzymes   c. BHAs
    b. AHAs   d. various seeds   _____

29. You can lighten and brighten skin color with these products:
    a. brighteners only
    b. lighteners only
    c. ceramides
    d. lighteners and brighteners   _____

30. Which of the following products should your clients apply without fail after an exfoliation service?
    a. moisturizer   c. sunscreen
    b. anti-irritant   d. foundation   _____

31. Antioxidants play this role in skin care:
    a. kill free radicals
    b. neutralize free radicals
    c. increase free radical activity
    d. encourage oxidation ____

32. Which ingredients help strengthen the immune system and stimulate the metabolism?
    a. polyglucans and beta-glucans
    b. glycoproteins
    c. peptides
    d. tissue respiratory factors ____

33. The functions of glycoproteins include:
    a. reducing the appearance of fine lines and wrinkles by stimulating collagen production
    b. providing anti-inflammatory and moisturizing properties
    c. enhancing cellular metabolism, which boosts oxygen uptake in the cell
    d. neutralizing free radicals before they attach themselves to the cell membrane and destroy the cell ____

34. Ingredients that improve the spreadability of formulations are called:
    a. delivery systems
    b. liposomes
    c. vehicles
    d. polymers ____

35. These specific chemical systems deliver ingredients to targeted tissues of the epidermis:
    a. delivery systems
    b. pilot systems
    c. molecule systems
    d. all answers ____

36. Closed, lipid bilayer spheres that encapsulate ingredients, target their delivery to specific tissues of the skin, and control their release, are called:
    a. polypeptides
    b. peptides
    c. polymers
    d. liposomes ____

37. Skin care products use vitamins, such as vitamins C and E, for their _____ properties.
    a. antioxidant
    b. free-radical oxidization
    c. sunscreen
    d. idebenone action ____

38. Sunscreens use these two types of ingredients:
    a. natural and botanical
    b. natural and chemical
    c. only chemicals ingredients
    d. only natural ingredients ____

39. Vitamin A:
    a. strengthens the immune system
    b. removes impaired cells
    c. stimulates cell repair
    d. is an anti-irritant
    ____

40. Retinoic acid _____ the skin.
    a. peels
    b. wrinkles
    c. soothes
    d. irritates acne in
    ____

41. The FDA regulates these important aspects of cosmetics:
    a. safety issues
    b. claims made for a product
    c. labeling issues
    d. all answers
    ____

42. When the skin becomes excessively red, or the client complains of burning, you should immediately:
    a. apply cool water
    b. stop the treatment
    c. apply warm water
    d. apply witch hazel
    ____

43. Performing a test patch is the best way to do what?
    a. test for product efficacy
    b. avoid allergic reactions
    c. determine the strength of the product
    d. all answers
    ____

44. Which of the products below is formed by a decomposition of oils or fats, is an excellent skin softener and humectant, and a very strong water binder?
    a. glycerine
    b. alum
    c. petroleum jelly
    d. parabens
    ____

45. Willow bark, wintergreen, and sweet birch are sources of which acid?
    a. salicylic acid
    b. tartaric acid
    c. malic acid
    d. lactic acid
    ____

46. Sulfur in skin care products:
    a. acts as an inorganic sunscreen that reflects UV rays
    b. reduces oil gland activity and dissolves the skin's dry, dead cells
    c. acts as an inorganic sunscreen that reflects UVA rays
    d. serves as a lubricant and perfume fixative
    ____

47. Which of the following is marine-based?
    a. allantoin
    b. azulene
    c. kojic acid
    d. algae
    ____

48. Which of these functions pertain to witch hazel?
    a. astringent
    b. antiseptic
    c. toning
    d. all answers
    ____

49. Aromatherapy treats the:
    a. mind
    b. body
    c. spirit
    d. all answers   _____

50. When you use plant extracts for therapeutic benefits, it is called:
    a. phytochemicals
    b. phytotherapy
    c. phtyochemistry
    d. phytoestrogen   _____

51. The sense of smell pertains to which system?
    a. olfactory system
    b. ocular system
    c. stereopsis system
    d. auditory system   _____

52. Vitamin C ester in skin care preparations stimulates:
    a. collagen degradation
    b. fibroblasts
    c. elastin degradation
    d. oxidation activity   _____

53. Identify the natural ingredients that can positively impact mature skin:
    a. green tea
    b. squalane oil
    c. dipotassium
    d. all answers   _____

54. DMAE (dimethylethanolamine):
    a. boosts the effects of nutrients
    b. boosts the effects of other antioxidants
    c. improves oxygen in the skin cells
    d. protects against infection   _____

55. What do topical ingredients need in order to most effectively treat the skin?
    a. chemicals
    b. natural ingredients
    c. AHAs
    d. high-tech delivery systems   _____

56. Which of the following represent categories of skin care?
    a. exfoliants and moisturizers
    b. toners, serums, and ampoules
    c. masks, sunscreens, and hydrators
    d. all answers   _____

57. When products are rinsed clean with water and do not strip the skin's natural acid mantle, they are considered ideal as:
    a. toners
    b. astringents
    c. cleansers
    d. exfoliants   _____

58. _____ are detergent-type foaming cleansers for oily skin.
   a. Cleansing gels
   b. Cleansing creams
   c. Cleansing lotions
   d. Cleansing gels and cleansing creams   _____

59. A product that is solely used to remove eye makeup or heavier makeup is called:
   a. toner   c. cleansing lotion
   b. cleansing gel   d. makeup remover   _____

60. What is the function of a freshener?
   a. restores the skin's natural pH after cleansing and hydrating the skin
   b. removes moisturizing products
   c. removes excess oil on the skin
   d. tones and tightens the skin   _____

61. Exfoliants improve:
   a. the skin's ability to retain moisture and lipids
   b. skin texture
   c. product penetration
   d. all answers   _____

62. Products that aid in extractions are called:
   a. toners   c. exfoliants
   b. astringents   d. fresheners   _____

63. Peeling off the top layers of the stratum corneum is done by a(n):
   a. mask   c. facial
   b. exfoliant   d. excoriation   _____

64. Contraindications for using harsh peeling techniques include:
   a. sensitive skin   c. acne-prone skin
   b. reactive skin   d. all answers   _____

65. Keratolytic enzymes:
   a. mechanically remove dead skin cells
   b. help speed up the breakdown of keratin
   c. inhibit keratin production
   d. remove blackheads   _____

66. Benefits derived from masks and packs include:
   a. hydrate   c. calm and soothe
   b. nourish   d. all answers   _____

67. The two types of masks are:
    a. hardening and softening   c. setting and non-setting
    b. hydrating and nourishing   d. clay and aloe   _____

68. Premature skin aging due to irritation occurs because:
    a. it doesn't cause premature aging
    b. it causes collagenase to breakdown collagen
    c. it increases the amount of hyaluronic acid
    d. it causes the development of cysts   _____

69. Masks that contain oils, emollients, and humectants are called:
    a. serum   c. clay
    b. non-setting   d. alginate   _____

70. Thermal masks containing gypsum are also called:
    a. custom-designed masks   c. clay masks
    b. paraffin wax masks   d. modelage masks   _____

71. Single applications of highly concentrated extracts in a water or
    oil base are called:
    a. ampoules   c. lipids
    b. serums   d. skin treatments   _____

72. Lotions, hydrators, and creams are all referred to as:
    a. antiaging products   c. humectants
    b. massage products   d. moisturizers   _____

73. UVA rays cause:
    a. sunscreen failure   c. skin aging
    b. skin rejuvenation   d. sunburn   _____

Part 4: Esthetics

CHAPTER 13—THE TREATMENT ROOM

1. Facial beds are also called:
    a. facial chairs
    b. esthetician's stools
    c. facial couches
    d. recliners
    ____

2. To ensure your physical well-being, a basic esthetician's stool must be:
    a. cushioned
    b. ergonomically correct
    c. on rollers
    d. customized
    ____

3. Another name for a hot towel warmer is:
    a. heater
    b. warm towel cabin
    c. steamer
    d. hot towel cabbie
    ____

4. The lamp that is used to analyze the skin and do detail work is called a:
    a. magnifying glass
    b. magnifying lamp
    c. lamp magnifier
    d. Wood's lamp
    ____

5. To assist clients in getting off the treatment bed, you need to have this piece of equipment:
    a. stairs
    b. step stool
    c. table extension
    d. escalator
    ____

6. The tools, supplies, and products you are using for a treatment are typically kept in a mobile:
    a. product cabinet
    b. utility cart
    c. cupboard
    d. shelf
    ____

7. Facial machines that are typically used during skin care services are:
    a. high-frequency machines
    b. brush machines
    c. vacuums and spray machines
    d. all answers
    ____

8. What is the function of an autoclave?
    a. produces galvanic current
    b. sterilizes equipment
    c. sanitizes equipment
    d. steams the face
    ____

9. What device heats wax and paraffin?
    a. paraffin bowl
    b. hot wax machine
    c. wax melter
    d. wax heater
    ____

10. Dispose of disposable lancets by placing them in a:
    a. sharps container   c. biohazard container
    b. lancet container   d. all answers   _____

11. What is the purpose of a dispensary?
    a. storing supplies
    b. mixing products
    c. a separate work space for preparing treatment products
    d. all answers   _____

12. Where are supplies stored?
    a. in clean, covered, labeled containers
    b. in open cupboards for easy access
    c. on open shelves for ease of inventory
    d. in unsealed bags   _____

13. Which of the following is not a supply?
    a. towel   c. client gown
    b. esthetician's stool   d. clean sheet   _____

14. _____ water is used in a facial steamer.
    a. Tap   c. Distilled
    b. Glacier   d. Bottled   _____

15. To support your clients' body during treatments, which items
    should you have on hand?
    a. a bolster for back support and a pillow or rolled hand towel
       for neck support
    b. a pillow to support the feet and a rolled hand towel or pillow
       for neck support
    c. a bolster for back support and arm rests to support the arms
    d. a pillow for neck support and a rolled towel for back support   _____

16. Never put a heated blanket under the bottom of the bed linens.
    Why?
    a. it will make clients thirsty
    b. it can become bunched midway through the treatment
    c. it will cause a higher sensitivity to products
    d. it is a fire hazard   _____

17. Products needed to perform a facial include:
    a. mask, exfoliant, and cleanser
    b. toner and face massage cream
    c. moisturizer, serum, and eye cream
    d. all answers   _____

68

18. Besides having a bolster or pillow available for clients, you should prepare the facial bed by:
    a. placing a blanket on top of the linens to keep the client warm.
    b. placing clean linens on the facial bed
    c. laying out one hand towel to be placed under the head
    d. all answers   _____

19. Which items/equipment should be heated before doing a basic facial?
    a. hot towel cabbie and towels
    b. face steamer and hot towel cabbie
    c. wax warmer and steamer
    d. none of these   _____

20. Before performing a facial, what should you do?
    a. rest for 10 minutes in order to be fresh for the service
    b. wash your hands with antibacterial soap
    c. wash your clients' hands with antibacterial soap
    d. wash your hands with bacterial soap   _____

21. Never place these items on a bare counter:
    a. clean supplies only   c. clean or dirty supplies
    b. dirty supplies only   d. equipment   _____

22. What should you explain to clients before they get on your treatment table?
    a. how to get on the table and where to position the head
    b. only how to get on the treatment table
    c. only where to position their head
    d. show clients where the restroom is located   _____

23. Why should a nail brush be on hand in your treatment room?
    a. to clean the nooks and crannies of your treatment room
    b. to clean your nails before performing services
    c. to clean the clients' nails before performing esthetic services
    d. to clean the clients' nails after performing esthetic services _____

24. When should you prepare all cotton cleansing pads, eye pads, and cotton compress pads that are used in a facial?
    a. before the service begins   c. two days in advance
    b. as you go   d. a week in advance   _____

25. After the _____, you should write up retail sales.
    a. consultation
    b. post-consultation
    c. service
    d. room is prepared for your next client   _____

26. These items must be placed in a sealable plastic bag and then in a covered waste container or biohazard container.
    a. gloves and extraction supplies
    b. soiled linens and towels
    c. disposable lancets
    d. all answers   _____

27. When giving a facial, treatment tools must be placed on surfaces that can be disposed of or _____.
    a. sterilized   c. disinfected
    b. sanitized   d. cleaned by hand   _____

28. What should you do before leaving work?
    a. prepare the room for the next day
    b. strip the room and prepare it the next day before your first client arrives
    c. leave the clean-up for the next morning, so the room is fresh for the first client of the day
    d. leave the clean-up for the next shift; it's their responsibility   _____

29. You should stock vinyl gloves in your treatment room because:
    a. they are more sanitary
    b. they are less likely to tear
    c. a client may be allergic to latex
    d. you may suddenly develop an allergic reaction to latex   _____

CHAPTER 14—BASIC FACIALS

1. Which of the following is the core treatment performed by estheticians?
   - a. waxing
   - b. facial
   - c. eyebrow shaping
   - d. facial massage
   _____

2. What is the goal of a facial?
   - a. improve and rejuvenate the skin
   - b. erase wrinkles
   - c. make fine lines disappear
   - d. permanently lift the skin
   _____

3. A medical office usually focuses on this type of treatment:
   - a. cleansing and toning
   - b. hydration
   - c. corrective
   - d. skin lightening
   _____

4. Facial benefits include:
   - a. deep cleansing
   - b. increases circulation and detoxifies
   - c. helps slow down premature aging
   - d. all answers
   _____

5. Making informed decisions for clients requires education in these areas:
   - a. skin analysis
   - b. skin care products
   - c. skin histology
   - d. all answers
   _____

6. Your success is _____ determined by how well you communicate with clients.
   - a. mainly
   - b. not
   - c. totally
   - d. partially
   _____

7. Retail sales is _____ of your job.
   - a. part
   - b. not part
   - c. sometimes part
   - d. the most important part
   _____

8. You can stay most informed and motivated by:
   - a. talking to coworkers
   - b. continuing your education
   - c. trying new products
   - d. reviewing your accomplishments
   _____

9. What should you do after consulting with your client?
   - a. assist them in preparing for the facial
   - b. put your client at ease
   - c. show them how to put on a facial wrap
   - d. show the client how to get on the treatment table safely
   _____

10. Which of the following answers is not one of the steps in performing a basic facial?
    a. cleansing
    b. microcurrent
    c. moisturizing
    d. extractions
    _____

11. You determine the products to be used in a facial by:
    a. consultation and skin analysis
    b. client questionnaire
    c. reading manufacturers' instructions
    d. clients' willingness to upgrade their services.
    _____

12. What should you be doing when analyzing the skin with a magnifying lamp?
    a. looking for obvious conditions and noting the skin type
    b. asking pertinent questions
    c. touching the skin
    d. all answers
    _____

13. In order to _____, warm, moist towels are applied prior to cleansing.
    a. warm and moisten the skin
    b. remove impurities
    c. tone the skin
    d. remove comedones
    _____

14. What should be done when product gets in a client's eyes during a service?
    a. client should flush her eyes with water
    b. you should flush the client's eyes with water
    c. wipe the client's eyes with tissues
    d. let the client's eyes naturally flush out the product
    _____

15. How do clay-lifting masks help the skin?
    a. moisturize
    b. exfoliate
    c. soothe
    d. smooth wrinkles
    _____

16. Warmth increases microcirculation, enhances product penetration, and:
    a. facilitates more effective extractions
    b. removes irritants
    c. minimizes pores
    d. reduces redness
    _____

17. When doing a deep pore cleansing, what do you use most often?
    a. moisturizing mask
    b. serum
    c. extra cleansing steps
    d. steam
    _____

18. Which of the following are desincrustation procedures?
    a. lifting masks   c. enzyme peels
    b. galvanic current   d. all answers   _____

19. If you apply improper pressure on a comedone, what can happen?
    a. it can make the follicular wall rupture
    b. the system may be poisoned
    c. cysts
    d. the blemish will be impossible to extract during subsequent visits   _____

20. Follicular walls that are perpendicular to the skin are located in
    these areas of the face:
    a. forehead and nose   c. jawline
    b. chin   d. all answers   _____

21. Besides tightening, toning, and hydrating the skin, certain masks can:
    a. relax the client
    b. reduce allergies
    c. draw impurities out of the pores
    d. all answers   _____

22. Daily application of a sunscreen is:
    a. optional
    b. imperative
    c. not necessary
    d. important during the summer months   _____

23. When are high-performance products most effective?
    a. at the end of a service
    b. at the beginning of a service
    c. any time during the service
    d. after the service   _____

24. As general rule, you should _____ when removing a
    product.
    a. rinse three times   c. rinse one time
    b. rinse two times   d. only use cotton pads   _____

25. What should you do before putting a warm, moist towel on a
    client's face?
    a. wring it out
    b. check the temperature to ensure it is not too hot or
       insufficiently heated
    c. make sure it is clean
    d. make sure it is in good shape   _____

26. When preparing to view your client's skin under the magnifying lamp, you should:
    a. allow your eyes to adjust to the magnified view of her skin
    b. cover the client's eyes with eye pads
    c. chat with your client to help her become more relaxed
    d. stretch to ensure you are comfortable while performing this phase of the service _____

27. What is the primary purpose(s) for viewing your client's skin under a magnifying source?
    a. determine skin type and condition
    b. determine how the skin has been treated in the past
    c. determine if the client sleeps in her makeup
    d. all answers _____

28. Approximately how far away should the facial steamer be when steaming the skin?
    a. 48"   c. 6"
    b. 18"   d. 36" _____

29. What should you do in front of your clients?
    a. wash your hands
    b. clean your room
    c. read instruction manuals
    d. refill your supplies _____

30. Which of the following should be covered during the post-consultation?
    a. retail products/home care
    b. skin care program
    c. current skin condition
    d. all answers _____

31. Why should you never put a lancet directly into the follicle?
    a. it can be painful and may damage the follicle
    b. it makes extractions impossible during subsequent visits
    c. it will cause scarring on the surface of the skin
    d. it will cause the comedone to seal _____

32. Dry skin may appear _____, but be _____ to the touch.
    a. flawless, bumpy   c. oily, dry
    b. youthful, old   d. fine, coarse _____

33. What type of product is necessary for dry skin?
    a. antiaging   c. greasy
    b. occlusive   d. non-occlusive _____

34. Which of the following factors can hasten skin aging?
    a. extreme climates, too much sun, wind, and salt water
    b. ill health and psychological problems
    c. extreme weight loss and environmental pollution
    d. all answers   ____

35. What should be placed on the skin prior to applying a gypsum/
    plaster mask?
    a. thin towel   c. gauze
    b. nothing   d. petroleum jelly   ____

36. Why is a thermal or paraffin mask beneficial to mature skin?
    a. plumps up skin and force feeds nutrients
    b. plumps up skin only
    c. forces the skin into a more youthful position
    d. erases fine lines   ____

37. When melting a paraffin mask product, it should be:
    a. 20°F hotter than body temperature
    b. a little more than body temperature
    c. 15°F hotter than body temperature
    d. body temperature   ____

38. Less steam and heat should be used on which skin type?
    a. sensitive   c. oily
    b. dry   d. normal   ____

39. When using an enzyme mask on sensitive skin it should be:
    a. formulated for sensitive skin
    b. formulated to remove dead skin cells
    c. diluted
    d. a premixed formulation   ____

40. Combination skin needs:
    a. cleansing creams   c. oil-based products
    b. emulsified products   d. water-based products   ____

41. How does benzoyl peroxide treat acne?
    a. sterilizes the follicle
    b. releases free radical oxygen that kills the bacteria
    c. irrigates and sloughs out acne impactions
    d. all answers   ____

42. Oil-free products are _____ non comedogenic.
    a. always   c. never
    b. not always   d. naturally   ____

43. Men often fail to take care of their skin because:
    a. it is unimportant   c. it is not masculine
    b. their minds are on business d. it is time consuming   ____

44. Pseudofolliculitis is the proper term for:
    a. face bumps   c. sun bumps
    b. razor bumps   d. hair bumps   ____

45. Hand movements during a man's facial should always:
    a. be firm   c. be light
    b. follow the hair growth   d. be aggressive   ____

CHAPTER 15—FACIAL MASSAGE

1. Which of the following describes massage?
   a. mechanical manipulation
   b. manual manipulation
   c. stimulates metabolism and circulation
   d. all answers
   _____

2. To do massage correctly and safely, you must have a thorough knowledge of:
   a. muscles
   b. nerves and blood vessels
   c. connective tissues
   d. all answers
   _____

3. Massage benefits include:
   a. reduces puffiness and sinus congestion
   b. aids in product absorption
   c. improves overall metabolism and activates sluggish skin
   d. all answers
   _____

4. A basic facial massage is performed for approximately:
   a. 10–15 minutes
   b. 30 minutes
   c. half of the facial time
   d. as long as the client wants you to massage her face
   _____

5. Your touch should be adjusted according to:
   a. how tense the client is feeling
   b. how energetic you feel
   c. client preference
   d. your preference
   _____

6. To properly massage the face, your hands must be:
   a. soft and sanitary
   b. free of artificial enhancements
   c. tough
   d. animated
   _____

7. Contraindications for facial massage include:
   a. rosacea
   b. inflamed acne
   c. sunburn
   d. all answers
   _____

8. The areas of the body that an esthetician can massage include:
   a. face, neck, and shoulders only
   b. face, neck, shoulders, and décolleté
   c. face, neck, shoulders, décolleté, and back
   d. face, neck, shoulders, and legs
   _____

9. Effleurage involves:
   a. wringing movements
   b. soft tapping movements
   c. firm, continuous stroking movements
   d. soft stroking movements _____

10. Pétrissage includes:
    a. pinching the skin with a light, firm pressure
    b. firm, circular movements
    c. tapping the skin
    d. soft, slow stroking _____

11. Fulling is a form of:
    a. friction   c. pétrissage
    b. wringing   d. effleurage _____

12. Massage involving a rubbing movement is called:
    a. fulling   c. chucking
    b. friction   d. lifting _____

13. Wringing and rolling are _____ movements.
    a. spreading out   c. tapotement
    b. pinching   d. pétrissage _____

14. Tapotement is also called:
    a. vibration   c. chucking
    b. percussion   d. Dr. Jacquet Movement _____

15. The therapist's body and shoulders are used to perform:
    a. tapotement   c. Dr. Jacquet Movement
    b. percussion   d. vibration _____

16. A basic male facial massage _____ involves movements that go against the growth of the beard.
    a. always   c. sometimes
    b. never   d. is lengthy and _____

17. Acupressure involves applying pressure:
    a. to specific points of the body
    b. to each muscle's insertion point
    c. on tense areas of the body
    d. to specific points on the feet and hands _____

18. Lymph drainage massage helps to:
    a. drain pus from comedones
    b. remove waste materials from the body
    c. drain lactic acid from muscle tissues
    d. improve elasticity in the skin _____

19. _____ is the key component of an aromatherapy massage.
    a. Massage lotion   c. Botanical-based cream
    b. Essential oil   d. all answers   _____

20. You can start a facial massage on the:
    a. chin   c. forehead
    b. décolleté   d. all answers   _____

21. What does a rhythmic flow promote?
    a. more effective results   c. well-being
    b. your style of massage   d. relaxation   _____

22. Massage movements are directed from the _____ to avoid muscle damage.
    a. insertion point toward the origin of the muscle
    b. insertion point to the mid-muscle
    c. origin of the muscle to the insertion point.
    d. mid-muscle to the insertion point   _____

23. Consecutively repeating all movements _____ times is a good rule of thumb.
    a. 3–6   c. 1–2
    b. 2–3   d. 4–6   _____

24. Which of the following are classical massage movements?
    a. effleurage and tapotement c. chucking and rolling
    b. petrissage and vibration   d. all answers   _____

CHAPTER 16—FACIAL MACHINES

1. Using electrical devices for therapeutic benefit is called:
   a. electrotherapy
   b. current therapy
   c. galvanic therapy
   d. direct current therapy
   _____

2. What does galvanic current do for the skin?
   a. moisturizes
   b. hydrates
   c. balances sebum production
   d. aids in penetration of products
   _____

3. The electric device that sanitizes the skin is called:
   a. ultrasound
   b. laser
   c. galvanic
   d. high-frequency
   _____

4. Valid contraindications for electrotherapy include:
   a. metal implants and pregnancy
   b. clients with epilepsy and other seizure disorders
   c. heart disease and pacemakers
   d. all answers
   _____

5. What is another name for a magnifying lamp?
   a. Wood's lamp
   b. loupe
   c. LED device
   d. magnifier
   _____

6. A magnifying lamp uses which type of bulb?
   a. halogen
   b. incandescent
   c. warm fluorescent
   d. fluorescent
   _____

7. The unit of measurement used for a magnifying lamp is a(n):
   a. ampere
   b. magnification power
   c. diopter
   d. voltage
   _____

8. The average magnifying lamp used by estheticians comes in values of 3-, 5-, and 10-diopter. What does this mean?
   a. 30, 50, and 100 times the power magnification
   b. 3, 5, and 10 times the power magnification
   c. each value describes the diameter of the various fluorescent bulbs
   d. 300, 500, and 1000 times the power magnification
   _____

9. A magnifying lens should be cleaned with:
   a. paper towels only
   b. a clean, soft cloth only
   c. a soft cloth and a disinfectant
   d. a clean treatment towel only
   _____

10. Pigmentation that is seen with a Wood's lamp is in the dermis and _____ lightened with professional skin care products.
    a. can be
    b. cannot be
    c. can sometimes be
    d. might be
    _____

11. A thick corneum layer appears as _____ when viewed through a Wood's lamp.
    a. light violet
    b. yellow or pink
    c. blue–white
    d. white fluorescence
    _____

12. Healthy skin appears _____ when viewed with a Wood's lamp:
    a. brown
    b. white fluorescence
    c. light violet
    d. blue–white
    _____

13. Hot towels provide _____ benefits.
    a. soothing
    b. softening
    c. warming
    d. all answers
    _____

14. A hot towel cabinet should be cleaned with disinfectant:
    a. once a day
    b. after each client
    c. every week
    d. twice a day
    _____

15. The primary purpose of the rotary brush is:
    a. extractions
    b. save your hands from doing too much during a service
    c. deeply exfoliates the skin
    d. lightly exfoliates the skin
    _____

16. What skin type(s) or conditions should not be treated with a rotary brush?
    a. dry
    b. combination
    c. oily
    d. inflamed
    _____

17. When using a rotary brush, it should be
    a. dripping wet
    b. damp
    c. dry
    d. saturated
    _____

18. Rotary brushes should be washed with:
    a. antibacterial soap only
    b. soap and water only
    c. soap and water and then immersed in a sanitizer
    d. soap and water and then immersed in a hospital-strength disinfectant
    _____

19. Every time you use a steamer, you should:
    a. sanitize the glass
    b. wipe down the outside of the glass with a high-level disinfectant
    c. make sure the rubber seal is clean
    d. refill with fresh distilled water   ____

20. Should you leave water in the steamer overnight?
    a. if there's enough water to do a few facials the next day
    b. never
    c. always
    d. depends on whether you are working the next day   ____

21. What product(s) should you use to clean the inside of the steamer jar?
    a. distilled water and white vinegar
    b. distilled water and apple cider vinegar
    c. hospital-strength disinfectant
    d. distilled water and hospital-strength disinfectant   ____

22. What can result from using tap water in your steamer?
    a. foul-smelling odor
    b. mineral deposits
    c. damage to your heating element
    d. scum buildup   ____

23. You should not use a suction device on:
    a. super sensitive skin   c. inflamed skin
    b. couperose skin   d. all answers   ____

24. The two significant reactions caused by galvanic current are:
    a. chemical and ionic
    b. ionic and manual
    c. chemical and mechanical
    d. desincrustation and chemical   ____

25. Galvanic current is used during desincrustation to create a chemical reaction that:
    a. liquefies the top layers of the stratum corneum
    b. disinfects acne pustules
    c. solidifies sebum
    d. emulsifies sebum   ____

26. What is placed on the skin's surface when performing a desincrustation?
    a. descaling solution
    b. alkaline-based electronegative solution
    c. sulfur mask
    d. alpha hydroxy acids   ____

27. People suffering from epilepsy or chronic migraines, or who are pregnant or wear braces:
    a. should not have a galvanic treatment
    b. should have a shortened galvanic service
    c. need a galvanic treatment every time they have a facial
    d. should only occasionally have a galvanic treatment _____

28. The most common desincrustation fluid used when performing anaphoresis is:
    a. baking soda and water
    b. salt and water
    c. vinegar and water
    d. apple cider vinegar _____

29. Which answer best explains iontophoresis?
    a. introduces water-soluble products without ions into the skin
    b. introduces insoluble products with ions into the skin
    c. introduces insoluble products without ions into the skin
    d. introduces water-soluble products with ions into the skin _____

30. Ionic penetration takes these two forms: cataphoresis and _____.
    a. anaphoresis
    b. iontophoresis
    c. ionization
    d. negative pole _____

31. An ionto mask uses galvanic current for:
    a. deep pore cleansing or penetration of product
    b. desincrustation
    c. blackhead extractions
    d. preventing product absorption _____

32. Which type of current is used by high-frequency machines?
    a. Tesla
    b. sinusoidal
    c. thermolysis
    d. single polarity _____

33. Does high frequency allow penetration of products into the skin?
    a. no
    b. yes
    c. if the frequency is high enough
    d. if there is an alternating current present _____

34. The benefits of using high frequency on a client's skin include:
    a. has an antiseptic effect and increases cell metabolism
    b. helps oxygenate the skin and stimulates circulation
    c. helps coagulate and heal open lesions after extractions and generates a warm feeling that has a relaxing effect on the skin
    d. all answers _____

35. The proper procedure for cleaning the glass electrode of a high-frequency machine includes:
    a. immersing the glass and metal in a disinfectant solution
    b. putting it in an ultraviolet cabinet
    c. immersing the glass portion in a disinfectant solution
    d. placing it in an autoclave   _____

36. What is the spray machine used for?
    a. removes all debris off the face after extractions
    b. removes remaining bits of mask
    c. firms the skin
    d. calms and hydrates the skin   _____

37. The Lucas sprayer was invented by:
    a. Dr. Louis Pasteur   c. Dr. Lucas Woods
    b. Dr. Marie Curie   d. Dr. Lucas Championniere   _____

38. Paraffin masks:
    a. balance oily skin   c. are clay masks
    b. hydrate dry skin   d. desensitize skin   _____

39. A crockpot shouldn't be used in lieu of a paraffin heater because:
    a. a paraffin heater makes your treatment look more professional
    b. a paraffin heater keeps the heated at a safe heat level
    c. it draws more electricity, making it more expensive in the long run
    d. it leaves the too cold to apply to the skin   _____

40. The greatest advantage of purchasing separate facial machines, rather than an all-in-one unit, is:
    a. it is cheaper
    b. if one machine breaks down, you can continue using the other machines while the broken one is being repaired
    c. the individual machines are superior in terms of quality and performance
    d. you do not have to memorize all the different functions at one time   _____

41. The greatest advantage of having an all-in-one facial machine is:
    a. the individual parts have more power
    b. it conveniently provides all functions you need in a much smaller space
    c. quality of the overall machine
    d. it is less complicated in terms of operating the machine   _____

CHAPTER 17—HAIR REMOVAL

1. What is trichology?
   a. the scientific study of hair removal
   b. the scientific study of hair care products
   c. the scientific study of hair and its diseases
   d. the scientific study of hair _____

2. The main structures of the hair below the surface of the skin are:
   a. follicle, bulb, and papilla   c. sebaceous glands
   b. arrector pili muscle   d. all answers _____

3. A hair follicle is a mass of epidermal cells extending down into the dermis and forming what?
   a. bulb   c. sac
   b. tube   d. pore _____

4. What is the other name for a pilosebaceous follicle?
   a. dermal papilla   c. hair bulb
   b. vellus hair   d. hair follicle _____

5. Strong, healthy hair receives adequate amounts of:
   a. vitamins   c. nutrients
   b. minerals   d. all answers _____

6. Hair growth is created by the activity of cells in the:
   a. stratum corneum   c. basal layer
   b. pores   d. dermis _____

7. What are the oil ducts or sebaceous glands that are attached to the follicle responsible for?
   a. lubricating the skin and hair   c. making the hair shiny
   b. lubricating just the skin   d. protecting sensitive skin _____

8. Hair found on a fetus is called:
   a. pre-birth hair   c. down
   b. peach fuzz   d. lanugo _____

9. Vellus is:
   a. telogen hair   c. anagen hair
   b. short, fine, downy hair   d. catagen hair _____

10. Hair growth occurs in these stages:
    a. anagen, catagen, and telogen   c. anagen and telogen
    b. catagen and telogen   d. catagen and anagen _____

11. Hair and skin are good barometers for what?
    a. state of a person's health
    b. state of mind
    c. attitude toward appearance
    d. lifestyle ____

12. Hirsutism is:
    a. hypertrichosis   c. baldness
    b. excessive hair growth   d. thin hair ____

13. The menopause moustache is caused by:
    a. estrogen   c. adrenocortical activity
    b. hormonal distress   d. cumulative sun exposure ____

14. The two types of hair removal are:
    a. deep and shallow   c. thinning and complete
    b. temporary and permanent d. anagen and catagen ____

15. Removing hair by using electricity is called:
    a. electrocoagulation   c. electrolysis
    b. laser   d. thermolysis ____

16. Galvanic, thermolysis, and blend are three methods of hair removal used by this method:
    a. electrolysis   c. IPL
    b. laser   d. photoepilation ____

17. IPLs:
    a. use quick flashes of light
    b. shatter the targeted hair bulb without allowing heat to build up and burn the surrounding skin
    c. reduce hair and spider veins
    d. all answers ____

18. What is depilation?
    a. removing the hair at the root
    b. removing the hair at or near the surface of the skin
    c. removing hair from the bottom of the follicle
    d. permanently removing the hair ____

19. What is epilation?
    a. removes hair from the bottom of the follicle
    b. removes hair by breaking contact between the bulb and the papilla
    c. pulls hair out of the follicle
    d. all answers ____

20. Folliculitis barbae is commonly called:
    a. baldness
    b. ingrown hair
    c. overgrowth of unhealthy hair
    d. patchy hair loss   _____

21. A product that removes hair is called:
    a. depilatory   c. depilation
    b. epilation   d. sugaring   _____

22. Which of the following answers accurately describes tweezing?
    a. using tweezers to pull hair out by the root one at a time
    b. using tweezers, thread, or sugar to pull out unwanted hair
    c. a faster method than waxing for hair removal
    d. permanently removing the hair by pulling it out, one hair
        at a time   _____

23. Which answer(s) best describes threading:
    a. uses 100% cotton thread
    b. thread is twisted and rolled along the surface of the skin
    c. entwines hair in the thread and lifts it out of the follicle
    d. all answers   _____

24. Waxing failures are caused by:
    a. skin that is not held taut
    b. wax has been used too many times
    c. fine hair
    d. hair is too long   _____

25. The two types of wax are:
    a. melted and solid   c. beads and disks
    b. hard and soft   d. blocks and pellets   _____

26. Common ingredients added to waxes are:
    a. azulene   c. tea tree oil
    b. chamomile   d. all answers   _____

27. Which of the following statement(s) accurately describe(s)
    hard waxes?
    a. gentle enough for the face
    b. strong enough to remove coarse hairs
    c. often preferred for the bikini area and underarms
    d. all answers   _____

28. Basic waxing supplies include:
    a. wax and warmer, cleansers, and pre- and post-epilation solutions
    b. muslin or pellon, thread, scissors, and cotton supplies
    c. gloves, disposable spatulas, tweezers, and gauze
    d. all answers ____

29. Wax that is water insoluble is removed by using a(n):
    a. water-soluble lotion
    b. oil-based solution
    c. warm water
    d. salt water ____

30. Which of the following best describes a roll-on wax?
    a. wax that is in an applicator and dispensed by a roll-on head
    b. wax that is dispensed from the wax warmer and rolled onto the skin
    c. a messy form of waxing that is not performed by estheticians
    d. a slow method for applying wax ____

31. When using oversize waxing strips:
    a. you can cover a larger area without compromising quality
    b. your waxing technique is compromised
    c. they are as safe as using appropriate-size strips
    d. they are preferred by most estheticians ____

32. Pellon is a:
    a. muslin
    b. linen
    c. fiber-like material that does not shed or stretch
    d. fiber-like material that is extremely stretchy ____

33. Which of the following answers best describe post-waxing materials?
    a. products with antiseptic and soothing properties and hair growth inhibitors
    b. products with antiseptic and soothing properties only
    c. hair growth inhibitors only
    d. products containing alcohol ____

34. When clients have these conditions and/or diseases, they should not receive a leg waxing service.
    a. phlebitis, varicose veins, or diabetes
    b. deep hair roots
    c. have only a few hairs
    d. are too hairy ____

35. You should never do a facial waxing on clients who have:
    a. sunburn, a history of fever blisters, pustules, or papules
    b. recent history of exfoliating topical medications such as Retin-A®
    c. recently used Accutane® or other acne medications or topical or oral cortisone
    d. all answers _____

36. Before any waxing service, you should:
    a. perform a consultation
    b. have a heart-to-heart chat about why the client wants a waxing service
    c. assess whether the hair growth is related to disease
    d. explain the extreme pain associated with waxing _____

37. Never apply wax over:
    a. warts, moles, abrasions, or inflamed skin
    b. freckles or birthmarks
    c. areas that have been waxed during previous appointments
    d. the fingers _____

38. Post-waxing precautions include:
    a. do not exfoliate for 48 hours
    b. avoid sun exposure for 48 hours
    c. avoid using creams with fragrance for 48 hours
    d. all answers _____

39. Which product is commonly used prior to a waxing service?
    a. witch hazel   c. alcohol
    b. aloe vera   d. cleansing lotion _____

40. What are the advantages of using powder prior to a waxing service?
    a. makes the hair more visible, helps protect the skin, and removes moisture
    b. prevents irritation
    c. talcum powder removes any excess moisture
    d. all answers _____

41. Strip (soft) waxing requires that you apply the wax:
    a. thickly
    b. against the direction of the hair growth
    c. in the direction of the hair growth
    d. in a horizontal direction _____

42. You should leave approximately a _____ margin on the pulling side of the fabric when doing a strip wax.
    a. 1"   c. 3"
    b. width of your palm   d. 2"

43. Hard wax should be applied how thick?
    a. the width of a dime
    b. the width of a quarter
    c. the width of a silver dollar
    d. the width of a nickel

44. When applying a muslin or pellon strip, what should you do?
    a. rub the strip in the opposite direction as the wax application
    b. rub the strip in the same direction as the wax application
    c. just stick it on there
    d. do not rub the strip

45. Properly shaped eyebrows are important because:
    a. they will make you look more intelligent
    b. they will look thicker
    c. correctly shaped eyebrows have a strong, positive impact on the overall attractiveness of the face
    d. they speak to style and fashion

46. Why should you apply a non-irritating antiseptic lotion after tweezing an area?
    a. relieves redness
    b. prevents infection and contracts the skin
    c. helps cover up any nicks you have caused by pinching the skin with the tweezers
    d. creates a better pull the next time you shape the brows

47. What should you do to minimize discomfort in sensitive areas during waxing?
    a. immediately place pressure on the waxed or tweezed area
    b. apply a numbing agent prior to the service
    c. blow on it
    d. give the client time to collect herself before continuing the service

48. What should you offer your client when doing a bikini service?
    a. disposable panties or a small, clean towel
    b. swimsuit bottom
    c. a napkin
    d. a tissue

49. The greatest challenge when waxing the armpits is:
    a. hair under the arms grows in several different directions
    b. armpits have different hair textures
    c. applying an even coat of wax
    d. all answers   ____

50. What should you take into account when waxing a man's back?
    a. the hair must be coarse
    b. the number of different growth patterns
    c. his threshold for pain
    d. how many waxing strips you need to cut   ____

CHAPTER 18—ADVANCED TOPICS AND TREATMENTS

1. Superficial peeling, exfoliation, keratolysis, and desquamation are terms for removing the excessive accumulation of dead cells from the:
    a. stratum corneum
    b. stratum spinosum
    c. stratum granulosum
    d. stratum lucidum
    ____

2. These products and methods are used to do light peels:
    a. manual scrubs
    b. microdermabrasion
    c. glycolic acid
    d. all answers
    ____

3. CRF (Cell Renewal Function) is influenced by:
    a. genetics, natural environment, and personal medical history
    b. lifestyle and personal care
    c. exfoliation methods
    d. all answers
    ____

4. TCA (trichloroacetic acid), glycolic acid (50% or more), and Jessner's peel (4–10 coats) are performed by:
    a. a physician
    b. an esthetician
    c. at home
    d. as part of a medical esthetician's private practice
    ____

5. To ensure a safe outcome with a peel, you should:
    a. always give a patch test 24–48 hours prior to a peel service to check for adverse reactions
    b. follow the manufacturer's directions
    c. consult with the client prior to applying a peel
    d. all answers
    ____

6. Glycolic acid:
    a. uses different percentages and pH factors to exfoliate the superficial layers of the epidermis
    b. is derived from sugar cane
    c. promotes superficial peeling
    d. all answers
    ____

7. Glycolic acid is frequently used for superficial peels because:
    a. it has the smallest molecular size of the AHA's
    b. it cannot effectively penetrate the epidermis
    c. it has the most balanced pH
    d. it has time-release properties
    ____

8. Salicylic acid is used to:
   a. correct dry skin
   b. treat acne
   c. treat couperose skin
   d. treat frequently peeled skin _____

9. The main qualities of salicylic acid are antiseptic and:
   a. inflammatory
   b. anti-inflammatory
   c. comedogenic
   d. deep peeling _____

10. A buffering product does what?
    a. prevents skin burns
    b. improves results
    c. reduces irritation
    d. reduces effectiveness _____

11. Light peels:
    a. improve the texture of the skin
    b. increase the cell renewal function (CRF)
    c. reduce the appearance of fine lines, wrinkles, and pigmentation
    d. all answers _____

12. When doing a consultation for a peel, you should:
    a. explain the procedures and realistic goals of the service
    b. show pictures of models with super-smooth skin
    c. show images of patients who have had medical-strength peels
    d. be optimistic when discussing your goals for the treatment _____

13. Identify the contraindications for performing a peel:
    a. acne scars and freckles
    b. oiliness and pore impactions
    c. herpes simplex and recent medical peels
    d. use of a different product line other than the one you recommend _____

14. These product ingredients are beneficial when combined with peels for mature and/or sensitive skin:
    a. ceramides, hyaluronic acid, phospholipids, and allantoin
    b. ascorbic acid and licorice root
    c. lactic acid and salicylic acid
    d. none of the above _____

15. Limitation of the strength of peels you are permitted to use in a salon is ultimately set by:
    a. peel strengths that are used by other estheticians in your area
    b. your regulatory agency
    c. your own judgment
    d. your client's desires with her skin _____

16. Why is it important to keep the skin hydrated after a peel?
    a. a peel robs the skin of much-needed sebum
    b. a peel temporarily creates a sluggish dermis
    c. a peel has a tendency to dry the skin
    d. a peel robs the skin of nutrients   _____

17. Microdermabrasion uses _____ exfoliation to lightly peel the skin.
    a. mechanical   c. aggressive
    b. electrical   d. gentle   _____

18. Which answer best describes microdermabrasion?
    a. powerful electronic vacuum
    b. sometimes abrades the skin with a hard applicator, such as a diamond tip
    c. usually sprays crystals on the face and then uses suction to vacuum them up and stimulate the skin
    d. all answers   _____

19. What does a successful microdermabrasion treatment depend on?
    a. proper use of the hand piece, rate of crystal flow, and vacuum setting
    b. length of the treatment
    c. quality of the crystals
    d. quality of the hand piece   _____

20. You should wear these items when cleaning up crystals:
    a. rubber gloves and mask
    b. gown and mask
    c. rubber gloves and goggles
    d. goggles and respirator   _____

21. Which of the following devices perform light therapies:
    a. lasers
    b. IPL (Intense Pulsed Light) systems
    c. LED (light-emitting diodes) devices
    d. all answers   _____

22. LED (Light-emitting diode) devices:
    a. use only white light   c. create skin sores
    b. operate at a very high energy   d. treat acne   _____

23. As we age, electrical impulses may _____ and cause skin aging.
    a. stop   c. become irregular
    b. speed up   d. slow   _____

24. When using a microcurrent device, the current is determined by the skin's _____.
    a. resistance
    b. ability to find a good rhythm
    c. cellular activity
    d. metabolism   _____

25. Ultrasound devices use:
    a. shallow sound waves
    b. a plastic spatula-like tool
    c. low-frequency mechanical oscillations
    d. deep-penetrating sound waves   _____

26. How does ultrasound benefit the skin?
    a. assists in product penetration
    b. uses a science called sonophoresis
    c. stimulates tissues and increases blood flow and oxygenation
    d. all answers   _____

27. Depending on the treatment product, body wraps can:
    a. remineralize the skin
    b. promote exfoliation
    c. congest skin tissues
    d. stimulate clients   _____

28. Body exfoliation services are synonymous with:
    a. body polishes and body glows
    b. peels
    c. smoothers
    d. all answers   _____

29. By using a combination of ingredients and _____, body scrubs can exfoliate and stimulate the skin.
    a. acids
    b. body cleansers
    c. patting
    d. friction   _____

30. One of the primary goals of clay, mud, and seaweed body masks is to:
    a. calm the skin
    b. polish the skin
    c. soften the skin
    d. remineralize the skin   _____

31. Which form(s) of water does hydrotherapy use?
    a. steam
    b. ice
    c. liquid
    d. all answers   _____

32. The core ingredients in balneotherapy are:
    a. mud and fango
    b. marine products such as algae
    c. botanical extracts
    d. essential oils   _____

33. Stone massage uses:
    a. only hot stones
    b. only cold stones
    c. stones heated to body temperature
    d. hot and cold stones   _____

34. Reflexology treats the whole body by applying pressure to:
    a. pressure points found throughout the body
    b. pressure points located on the feet and hands
    c. acupressure points throughout the body
    d. trigger points throughout the body ____

35. What are the three Ayurveda doshas?
    a. kapha, vatta, and delpha   c. pitta, kapha, and vatta
    b. vatta, delpha, and pitta   d. pitta, kapha, and alpha ____

36. The primary purpose of endermology is to:
    a. tighten sagging skin
    b. treat cellulite
    c. treat fat anywhere in the body
    d. all answers ____

37. Identify the primary benefit of manual lymph drainage:
    a. improves blood flow to the extremities
    b. warms the body
    c. stimulates blood flow throughout the lymphatic vessels
    d. stimulates the flow of lymph fluid through the lymphatic
       vessels ____

38. Medical aestheticians can be certified as:
    a. Certified Medical Aestheticians
    b. Physician's Assistants (PAs)
    c. Superior Estheticians
    d. Master Aestheticians ____

39. Non-ablative laser treatments:
    a. only remove the top layers of the epidermis
    b. do not remove tissue
    c. remove tissue
    d. do not treat wrinkles ____

40. Non-ablative intense pulsed light therapies (IPLs):
    a. cut through the epidermis to treat hyperpigmentation
       in the dermis
    b. remove warts
    c. bypass the epidermis to stimulate collagen in the dermis
       for wrinkle reduction
    d. remove tattoos ____

41. Botox® and dermal fillers are:
    a. harmful   c. prostheses
    b. silicone implants d. injectables ____

42. How does Botox® (botulinum toxin) work to reduce the
    appearance of lines and wrinkles?
    a. creates a temporary paralysis or diminished movement by
       blocking neurotransmitters
    b. has an ablative action
    c. prompts collagen production
    d. prompts elastin production   _____

43. Dermal fillers work best when:
    a. a variety of fillers are used in a single site
    b. patients have additional dermal fillers on a monthly basis
    c. used in conjunction with Botox®
    d. are derived from animal sources   _____

44. In medical jargon, a face lift is called a:
    a. rhinoplasty
    b. transconjunctival blepharoplasty
    c. blepharoplasty
    d. rhytidectomy   _____

45. Sclerotherapy involves:
    a. TCA (trichloroacetic acid) peels
    b. minimizing varicose veins
    c. laser resurfacing
    d. dermabrasion   _____

46. What does a clinical esthetician do?
    a. performs post-surgery facials
    b. works in a medical setting
    c. performs procedures such as mild peels
    d. all answers   _____

CHAPTER 19—THE WORLD OF MAKEUP

1. The primary goal of makeup is to:
   a. make small eyes bigger
   b. hide blotchy complexions
   c. give some color to the face
   d. enhance the natural beauty of the client   _____

2. Which of the following should you determine during a makeup consultation?
   a. lifestyle and preferences
   b. hair and eye color
   c. natural skin tone and face shape
   d. all answers   _____

3. Makeup artists must know how to _____ facial features.
   a. analyze   c. accentuate pleasing
   b. balance   d. all answers   _____

4. When choosing a makeup line, which of the following is most important?
   a. quality   c. price
   b. selection   d. packaging   _____

5. Foundation:
   a. allows women to change the color of their skin
   b. protects the skin from the outside elements
   c. hydrates
   d. moisturizes   _____

6. Dry skin is best suited for which formulation?
   a. water-based   c. oil-based
   b. oil-free   d. oil-in-water   _____

7. Water, stearic acid, cetyl alcohol, mineral oil, propylene glycol, lanolin derivatives, and insoluble pigments are commonly included in which type of makeup?
   a. mascara   c. foundation
   b. eye shadow   d. lip gloss   _____

8. Thicker foundation that gives heavier coverage is a(n):
   a. oil-and-powder foundation
   b. oil-based foundation
   c. mineral foundation
   d. cream foundation   _____

9. What mineral/sunscreen ingredient is commonly used in mineral makeup products?
   a. titanium dioxide
   b. tourmaline
   c. aluminum
   d. talc
   _____

10. A(n) _____ is created by foundation.
    a. blank canvas
    b. even canvas
    c. colored canvas
    d. smooth canvas
    _____

11. Remove concealer out of its container with (a):
    a. your fingers
    b. your client's fingers
    c. spatula
    d. makeup brush
    _____

12. Makeup for the cheeks is available in:
    a. cream
    b. liquid
    c. pressed (dry) and loose
    d. all answers
    _____

13. The primary purpose of eye shadow is to:
    a. contour and accentuate the eyes
    b. hide uneven skin tones on the eyelids
    c. balance the eyes with the brows
    d. create a total look
    _____

14. When you match eye shadow color to eye color, what does it do?
    a. creates a more natural look
    b. provides a classic look
    c. creates a flat field of color
    d. makes the eyes appear brighter and more expressive
    _____

15. Contrasting colors that _____ the eye color can enhance the eyes.
    a. are brighter than
    b. clash with
    c. compliment
    d. complement
    _____

16. The natural color of the iris appear(s) _____ when you use a darker color.
    a. darker
    b. lighter
    c. whiter
    d. invisible
    _____

17. What is an eye shadow called when it is lighter than the client's skin tone?
    a. base
    b. highlighter
    c. contour
    d. dark
    _____

18. When you are preparing to apply eye shadow, you should:
    a. remove the eye color with a spatula
    b. load up the brush with color
    c. sell the eye shadow to the client, and then apply it with her brush
    d. put on your own makeup ____

19. The eyebrows _____ the eyes.
    a. diminish the appearance of   c. upstage
    b. enlarge the appearance of   d. frame ____

20. When applying mascara, you should:
    a. use the wand from your client's mascara
    b. have your clients apply their own mascara
    c. use a disposable wand
    d. ask the client to gently close her eyes ____

21. At what point in the application should you use an eyelash curler?
    a. before you apply mascara
    b. after you apply mascara
    c. before or after applying mascara
    d. after you apply lipstick ____

22. What are paraffin, beeswax, carnauba, and candelilla?
    a. waxes that are never used in lipsticks
    b. waxes that are commonly used in lipsticks
    c. oils
    d. substances that have been banned by the FDA ____

23. Natural colorant(s) used in lipsticks include:
    a. iron oxides   c. annatto
    b. mica   d. all answers ____

24. What is the purpose of using a lip pencil?
    a. prevents feathering   c. adds definition
    b. ensures the proper shape   d. all answers ____

25. A brush with a firm, thin, angled bristle that is used on the eyebrows, or for eyeliner, is called a(n):
    a. angle brush   c. lash-and-brow brush
    b. fluff brush   d. eye shadow brush ____

26. What is the purpose of a firm eye shadow brush?
    a. gives you confidence
    b. blends eye shadow colors
    c. more suitable for lighter colors
    d. deposits dense color on the eyelids ____

27. To clean your makeup brushes, you should use:
    a. gentle shampoo
    b. spray-on sanitizer
    c. brush solvent
    d. all answers   _____

28. Primary colors:
    a. are generally used by a novice makeup artist
    b. cannot be obtained from a mixture of colors
    c. include red, yellow, and green
    d. include orange, violet, and blue   _____

29. What do you mix to form tertiary colors?
    a. equal amounts of a secondary color and its neighboring
       primary color
    b. equal parts of primary colors
    c. any three colors
    d. three secondary colors   _____

30. When complementary colors are placed next to each other, they:
    a. create a soft, neutral effect
    b. turn into pastels
    c. have a gray appearance
    d. appear brighter   _____

31. Cool colors have a _____ undertone.
    a. blue
    b. green
    c. violet or blue–red
    d. all answers   _____

32. Pink tones are not flattering on this skin color:
    a. ashen
    b. ruddy
    c. pale ivory
    d. olive   _____

33. Purple is not a good color choice for:
    a. warm skin tones
    b. pale skin tones
    c. reddish skin tones
    d. cool skin tones   _____

34. Black and white:
    a. combine well only with each other
    b. combine well with all colors
    c. combine poorly with light colors
    d. combine well with dark colors   _____

35. A neutral skin tone contains:
    a. equal amounts of warm and cool
    b. two parts warm to one part cool
    c. one part warm to two parts cool
    d. mostly cool   _____

36. When determining the perfect foundation, you should first:
    a. ask your client to pick out her favorite foundation colors
    b. ask your client if she likes to wear foundation every day
    c. determine if your client has a light, medium, or dark skin level
    d. assess whether your client has a warm or cool skin tone ____

37. Dark colors appear most subtle on:
    a. medium skin tones   c. a person wearing black
    b. dark skin tones   d. light skin tones ____

38. What should makeup do for your client?
    a. add a festive touch
    b. maximize good features and minimize less attractive features
    c. only maximize good features
    d. give her a dramatic look ____

39. When the face is widest at the temple and forehead, tapering
    down to the chin, it is a(n) _____ shape.
    a. oval   c. diamond
    b. square   d. round ____

40. A receding chin can be made to look more prominent by:
    a. making the chin the same color as the rest of the face
    b. using a lighter foundation on the chin
    c. there is nothing that you can do to visually correct a
       receding chin
    d. applying a darker shade on the chin to make it stand out ____

41. You can visually correct a wide nose by:
    a. placing a darker shade of foundation on both sides of the
       nose and a lighter shade on the center of the nose
    b. applying two coats of powder
    c. applying a darker foundation to the center of the nose
    d. avoiding foundation on the nose ____

42. When a client has close-set eyes:
    a. they are closer together than the length of both eyes
    b. they are closer together than the length of one eye
    c. they have a beady appearance
    d. they are less than one inch apart ____

43. You can make small eyes appear larger by:
    a. applying the shadow to the inner side toward the nose
    b. using the lightest color on the crease
    c. applying a dark shadow over the eyelids
    d. extending the eye shadow slightly beyond the eyes toward
       the temples ____

44. Overtweezing the brows can:
    a. make the brow look protruding   c. make the face look puffy
    b. create a surprised look   d. all answers   _____

45. What is the first thing you should do when correcting or shaping
    an eyebrow?
    a. remove all unnecessary hairs
    b. match the client's brows with the proper template
    c. turn the client away from the mirror
    d. start in the middle   _____

46. Creating the ideal eyebrow shape involves:
    a. measuring the inner corner of the eye upward
    b. measuring from the outer corner of the nose to the outer
       corner of the eye
    c. measuring from the outer circle of the iris of the eye upward
       while the client is looking straight ahead
    d. all answers   _____

47. What should you do to make large lips appear smaller?
    a. outline both the upper and lower lips and fill in with a
       frosted lipstick
    b. outline the upper and lower lips with a soft color to create a
       balanced outline
    c. build the corners of the mouth
    d. draw a thin line just inside the natural lip line, using a soft,
       flat color   _____

48. During your makeup consultation you should:
    a. visually assess the client's personal style and determine
       her skin type
    b. ask the client how many eye shadows she can buy
    c. ask the client about her favorite makeup brand
    d. ask the client how many shadows she has in her drawer at home   _____

49. You must perform your makeup applications in a:
    a. spacious area that reflects the quality of your makeup line
    b. neat and organized area
    c. front area of the salon
    d. all answers   _____

50. Disinfecting a makeup pencil involves:
    a. sharpening the pencil with a clean sharpener
    b. wiping off the tip with a clean tissue
    c. spraying the pencil with disinfectant
    d. sharpening the pencil with a clean sharpener, spraying with
       disinfectant, and then wiping with a clean tissue   _____

51. Sponges are good for:
    a. wiping off mascara spots
    b. blending foundation only
    c. blending concealer only
    d. blending foundation, concealer, and powder _____

52. Where should you distribute your products after selecting your colors and foundation?
    a. individual cups
    b. artist's pallet
    c. paper towel
    d. aluminum foil _____

53. The client's skin should not be gently lifted or manipulated during the makeup application because:
    a. it causes permanent wrinkles
    b. it starts the wrinkling process
    c. it will change the look when you let go of the skin
    d. it treats the skin roughly _____

54. You should apply this makeup product first:
    a. concealer
    b. foundation
    c. mascara
    d. eye shadow _____

55. Important question(s) to ask clients prior to a makeup application include:
    a. Do you wear contact lenses?
    b. Do you have allergies?
    c. How much makeup do you normally wear?
    d. all answers _____

56. Before applying makeup you should:
    a. make up a face chart
    b. wash your hands
    c. show the client your license
    d. rest _____

57. Where should clients look while you are applying mascara?
    a. look straight ahead
    b. look to the side
    c. look at a fixed point
    d. close their eyes _____

58. For special occasions involving subdued lighting, you should:
    a. apply a light amount of makeup
    b. apply a heavy amount of makeup
    c. use brighter colors
    d. apply more definition to the eyes, lips, and cheeks _____

59. For a special occasion, most clients prefer:
    a. heavy makeup
    b. brighter or darker colors
    c. more eyeliner
    d. the same makeup they wear every day   _____

60. Band lashes are:
    a. individual lashes   c. eyelashes on a strip
    b. a clump of lashes   d. high fashion   _____

61. Place an eyelash strip:
    a. on the lash line
    b. on the skin just above the lash line
    c. on the natural eyelashes
    d. anywhere you please   _____

62. Eyelash adhesive:
    a. is hyperallergenic   c. is allergenic
    b. is non-allergenic   d. can be allergenic   _____

63. What is the best way to remove artificial eyelashes?
    a. with tweezers
    b. ask the client to remove them prior to her appointment
    c. use pads saturated with a special solution
    d. let them fall off naturally   _____

64. When applying eyelashes, first:
    a. brush the eyelashes to ensure they are clean and free of
       foreign matter
    b. apply a thin band of adhesive
    c. wash the eyelashes with face cleanser
    d. apply witch hazel   _____

65. Tinting the lashes and brows involves:
    a. lightening or darkening the lashes and brows
    b. darkening the lashes and brows
    c. bleaching the hairs
    d. all answers   _____

66. When tinting the lower lashes, applying cream and a pad under
    the eye is important for this reason:
    a. it prevents tint from bleeding onto the skin
    b. it enables the tint to better penetrate the lashes
    c. it makes your service look more professional
    d. it is regulated by state board   _____

67. What are lash extensions?
    a. clumps of eyelashes
    b. individual lashes that are applied one by one to the client's natural lashes
    c. the same thing as strip lashes
    d. lashes made of animal hair ____

68. Permanent cosmetic tattooing is also called:
    a. eye shadow tattooing
    b. temporary makeup
    c. permanent makeup
    d. macropigmentation ____

69. Who performs permanent makeup services?
    a. tattoo artists
    b. estheticians
    c. medical technicians
    d. all answers ____

70. The advantages of airbrush makeup include:
    a. hygienic, long-lasting, and rub and water resistant
    b. more efficient and faster to apply
    c. lightweight, natural, and flawless looking
    d. all answers ____

71. Makeup airbrushing includes:
    a. face, nail, and body art
    b. nail polish applications
    c. skin care
    d. photo touch-ups ____

Part 5: Business Skills

CHAPTER 20—CAREER PLANNING

1. Being a good student means you are:
   a. an outgoing student
   b. an active studier
   c. willing to put in your time
   d. a natural skin care expert   ____

2. Before your State Board test, it is all right to feel:
   a. some anxiety
   b. that you will fail the first time
   c. an unpleasant experience is about to take place
   d. all answers   ____

3. Deductive reasoning used in testing includes:
   a. watching for grammatical clues
   b. studying the stem
   c. eliminating answers that you know are wrong
   d. all answers   ____

4. When interviewing for your first esthetics position, showcase your
   best qualities by defining:
   a. personal skills and qualities that make you a desirable
      employee
   b. personal interests that would make you a well-rounded
      employee
   c. the product lines that you want to use for services
   d. your dream salon   ____

5. Identify the treatments commonly performed by an independent
   skin care clinic or day spa:
   a. deep skin peels
   b. antiaging facials
   c. laser hair removal
   d. hyperpigmentation in the dermis   ____

6. A full-service salon always provides:
   a. hair, nail, and skin care services
   b. fitness programs
   c. specialty services
   d. services that do not pertain to beauty and well-being   ____

7. Medical spas operate within:
   a. hospitals
   b. medical practices
   c. cosmetic surgery offices
   d. all answers _____

8. Which answer best describes a resort spa?
   a. superior to day spas
   b. inferior to day spas
   c. all-inclusive spa retreats
   d. fat farms _____

9. What is the focus of a wellness spa?
   a. treating non-specific diseases
   b. maintaining optimal health
   c. super-relaxing experiences
   d. all answers _____

10. A booth rental establishment involves:
    a. leasing a room to provide services independently
    b. a co-op
    c. leasing the entire salon
    d. paying commission on services rendered _____

11. A résumé should include:
    a. summary of education
    b. summary of work experience
    c. accomplishments and achievements
    d. all answers _____

12. Your résumé should:
    a. use clear, concise language
    b. use vivid descriptions of your qualifications
    c. highlight your attitude
    d. outline certain work conditions _____

13. It is important to stress your_____ in your résumé.
    a. salary expectations
    b. transferable skills
    c. hobbies
    d. family life _____

14. A cover letter to a résumé should begin with:
    a. your license number
    b. a list of the certifications you have earned
    c. position of interest
    d. personal references _____

15. In addition to your résumé and cover letter, you may want to
    prepare a portfolio that includes:
    a. before-and-after photos relating to skin care or makeup artistry
    b. letters of recognition for community service or volunteer work
    c. award certificates
    d. all answers _____

16. Before accepting your first position as an esthetician, you should:
    a. find out as much as possible about the salon's history and philosophy
    b. meet every person who works at the salon
    c. count the number of stations vs. the number of treatment rooms
    d. take more classes ____

17. To assess whether or not a job is right for you, you should ask yourself:
    a. What support will I need to ensure my success?
    b. Am I in agreement with the salon or spa's philosophy?
    c. What is the most important consideration for me in terms of work conditions?
    d. all answers ____

18. Franchise salons or spas:
    a. are independent salons
    b. have no more than five locations
    c. are owned by individuals, but are still part of a larger organization or chain
    d. are chain salons ____

19. It is advisable to visit salons or spas:
    a. before you graduate
    b. as soon as you graduate
    c. after you take your licensure test
    d. as soon as you receive your license ____

20. During an information interview, it is recommended to ask about:
    a. the duties and responsibilities required by the estheticians on staff
    b. if the salon is always busy
    c. if the clients make enough money to afford esthetic services
    d. if the staff will support your services ____

21. You can network by:
    a. joining professional organizations
    b. attending industry trade shows and educational seminars
    c. requesting an interview with the who's who of skin care in your area, whether it's by phone, e-mail, or in person
    d. all answers ____

22. When interviewing:
    a. your skin should reflect healthy skin care practices
    b. you should wear intricate makeup
    c. you should note how the stylists dress
    d. you should broadly smile at all times ____

23. Answering these question(s) during your interview should be expected:
    a. What is your approach to customer service?
    b. How do you feel about promoting retail sales?
    c. What are your long-term career goals?
    d. all answers   _____

24. You can become part of your salon's goal to have a productive business by:
    a. keeping a schedule that benefits the salon's clients
    b. following a set schedule
    c. creating your own protocols
    d. creating your own standards   _____

25. What is included in employment guidelines?
    a. detailed job description highlighting specific duties and responsibilities
    b. commission that each esthetician makes on staff
    c. your preferred products
    d. which organizations you may, or may not, join   _____

26. As a skin care professional, you should:
    a. frame your license so it is more noticeable to clients
    b. investigate new products and techniques
    c. stay with the same protocols because they work
    d. only support your favorite products because you are confident that they work   _____

27. An employee evaluation includes:
    a. feedback and assessment of retail and service sales
    b. whether or not you are meeting your job requirements
    c. your attitude
    d. all answers   _____

28. Tips:
    a. are not taxable
    b. are considered additional income by the IRS
    c. are shared with the owner
    d. represent the majority of your income   _____

CHAPTER 21—THE SKIN CARE BUSINESS

1. What should you have before going into business for yourself?
   a. clear vision and good business skills
   b. some real, practical experience in the skin care business and a strong commitment
   c. energy
   d. all answers ____

2. Managing day-to-day operations requires:
   a. client recommendations
   b. knowing instantly which products you should include in your practice
   c. solving problems on a regular basis
   d. all answers ____

3. What are booth renters responsible for?
   a. building and managing their own clients, purchasing supplies, and keeping records
   b. making all business decisions without consulting with the salon owner
   c. doing complimentary services for the salon owner
   d. buying their own supplies, only ____

4. Before becoming a booth renter, it is vital to:
   a. investigate the legality of the situation
   b. see if booth renters are accepted by the esthetics community in your area
   c. find the least expensive rent and products available, to ensure that you can pay your overhead
   d. plan for weeks you will be short on cash by asking for rent leniency ____

5. _____ states require a special license for booth renters.
   a. No   c. Some
   b. The majority of   d. All ____

6. Who should you target when you are planning to offer high-end services?
   a. wealthy clients who can afford these services
   b. high-end clients who can afford these services
   c. family-oriented areas
   d. new areas ____

7. Identify one of the many important factors you should consider when scouting for a location:
   a. find areas that have no competition
   b. find areas that have a lot of competition as this shows signs of a lucrative market
   c. find areas that have a moderate number of salons offering skin care
   d. ignore the competition; your skills and services stand on their own ____

8. What should a business plan include?
   a. detailed description of your business and all costs related to operations
   b. media sources that are willing to trade services
   c. previous work history and personal qualities that will make you successful
   d. cost-cutting measures in case you do not meet your monetary goals ____

9. As a salon owner, your insurance needs include:
   a. liability and malpractice
   b. disability and burglary
   c. theft and business interruption
   d. all answers ____

10. When there are two or more owners involved in a salon, what is it called?
    a. joint venture   c. partnership
    b. corporation   d. sole proprietorship ____

11. Which of the following are benefits of a partnership?
    a. increased capital for investment
    b. greater pool of skills and talent to draw from
    c. someone to share the work and decision-making responsibilities
    d. all answers ____

12. A corporation is managed by:
    a. a sole proprietor   c. a board of directors
    b. partners   d. a corporate family ____

13. It is essential to seek the advice of _____ before purchasing an existing business.
    a. your former teachers
    b. an accountant and business lawyer
    c. friends who have owned businesses
    d. people you respect ____

14. Why is having a security checklist important?
    a. so the fire department will know where your fire extinguishers are located
    b. to properly balance the cash register
    c. to ensure that those responsible for closing or opening the salon are aware of what it entails to safely do so
    d. so the police will know the code to your burglar alarm   _____

15. What determines the amount of capital needed to operate your business for two years?
    a. business ledger
    b. business plan
    c. accounting program
    d. gross receipts   _____

16. What must you learn to do with your staff in order to be a successful manager?
    a. work cooperatively
    b. micromanage
    c. make allowances for bad behavior
    d. encourage them to love their job   _____

17. Day-to-day accounting practices provide:
    a. gross income and the cost of operations
    b. net income
    c. just gross income
    d. net profit   _____

18. Consumption supplies are:
    a. supplies used to conduct business operations on a daily basis
    b. retail products
    c. things like toilet paper, paper towels and cotton, only
    d. all answers   _____

19. What quality is shared by most successful owners?
    a. willingness to sacrifice, no matter how hard it might be
    b. willingness to work hard
    c. luck
    d. being crafty   _____

20. When laying out your space, it is essential that:
    a. it provides maximum efficiency
    b. every area has ample space
    c. the salon reception desk is within 10 feet of the entrance
    d. you have natural lighting   _____

21. You can maximize your efforts when looking for potential employees by:
    a. developing a list of questions and criteria for evaluating prospective employees
    b. not being too specific
    c. knowing what you want, but be willing to settle for less
    d. all answers

22. You can create the best work environment in terms of productivity and stability by:
    a. setting rigid guidelines and sticking to them
    b. letting your employees help you set the guidelines for your salon
    c. being lenient and always seeing the best in people
    d. setting sensible rules and directions

23. As an employer, it is important to:
    a. always arrive early and leave late
    b. do fewer client services and more employee supervision
    c. work harder than your employees
    d. set clear goals and objectives and be consistent

24. Being a good staff manager includes:
    a. acting decisively and not letting situations linger
    b. learning to expect the best
    c. showing leadership
    d. all answers

25. What is most important to build with clients?
    a. trusting relationships
    b. intuitive relationships
    c. friendly rapport
    d. happy conversations

26. A receptionist should possess:
    a. excellent interpersonal communication and public relations skills
    b. good accounting skills
    c. a good sense of fashion and makeup
    d. an excellent gift of the gab

27. Confirming appointments is most important because it:
    a. keeps business flowing smoothly
    b. looks professional in the eyes of the clients
    c. helps you determine in advance what you will make that day
    d. promotes customer satisfaction with your services

28. What is the best way to handle phone messages during the course of a busy day?
    a. return messages as soon as possible
    b. wait until the end of the day when things are quiet and you can give your callers all your attention
    c. call in the morning when people are fresh
    d. return calls immediately, even if it means that you must pull away from a client
                                                                    _____

29. What does public relations entail?
    a. handing out coupons to clients every time they come to visit your salon
    b. bragging about your services and products
    c. frequent advertising
    d. building a reputation for quality service and fair business practices
                                                                    _____

CHAPTER 22—SELLING PRODUCTS AND SERVICES

1. Retail in a salon situation is:
   a. a secondary objective
   b. a fundamental objective
   c. an added bonus
   d. is not important
   ____

2. Which answer most adequately describes retailing in a salon setting?
   a. not pleasant, but should be done anyway
   b. a necessary and reputable part of your work
   c. the bane of your work
   d. at the core of your services
   ____

3. To be successful in retail sales, you must be:
   a. a natural salesperson
   b. motivated and committed to products' value
   c. skilled in sales techniques
   d. all answers
   ____

4. Skin care clients:
   a. look to you for guidance in recommending skin care products
   b. prefer to shop in drugstores where products cost a fraction of the cost of professional skin care products
   c. still believe in soap and water, and it is your job to convert them
   d. have no budget when it comes to taking care of their skin
   ____

5. To successfully retail to clients, you should:
   a. position products as genuine solutions to problems
   b. demonstrate the products like salespeople in department stores
   c. bag the products and present the client with a receipt before discussing the products
   d. all answers
   ____

6. When presenting products to a client, you must:
   a. understand the manufacturer's philosophy
   b. understand the key ingredients in the product
   c. be able to convey the benefits to the client
   d. all answers
   ____

7. Successfully recommending a product to a client must include:
   a. using the product yourself
   b. admiring the packaging
   c. believing in the product
   d. maintaining an ample retail stock
   ____

8. Why does the client questionnaire provide valuable information about retailing?
   a. it lists the client's habits and goals
   b. it lists the client's vulnerabilities
   c. it gives clues about the client's views of professional products
   d. all answers ____

9. Estheticians who are successful at retailing keep abreast of:
   a. unethical practices by competitors
   b. drug store promotions
   c. promises made by competitors
   d. different products and techniques that are currently on the market ____

10. Identify the answer that best describes marketing in a salon situation:
    a. strategies for how goods and services are bought, sold, or exchanged
    b. promotional events
    c. advertising campaigns
    d. sales meetings ____

11. A limited sales promotion is:
    a. limited to a single esthetician on staff
    b. products sold at a discount on slower times of the week
    c. held for a limited time
    d. sold in only one area of the salon ____

12. A new client gives you the opportunity to:
    a. take her on a tour of the salon
    b. make a product presentation
    c. make a good first impression
    d. all answers ____

13. Salons are kept going by:
    a. attracting new clients
    b. retaining clients
    c. posters and other marketing displays in the salon
    d. frequent menu changes ____

14. What supports a steady stream of business?
    a. providing clients with your undivided attention
    b. being efficient in how you do your services
    c. providing good customer service
    d. all answers ____

15. The growth of your business should be supported by:
    a. talking about skin conditions in the employee's lounge
    b. keeping staff abreast of new services
    c. being interested in learning about hair in order to connect with stylists
    d. wearing more colorful smocks   _____

16. Identify the answer that accurately describes a prescriptive memo:
    a. a form that provides the names and numbers of dermatologists whom you admire
    b. ingredients of key products
    c. retail products that you recommend for home care
    d. a list of products prescribed by physicians   _____

17. Why do you make follow-up phone calls to clients?
    a. to allay your fears regarding the quality of your services
    b. to ensure that clients are doing well post-service and with their home-care regimen
    c. don't do it; it will concern clients
    d. to help you talk more about the quality of your retail products   _____

Part 1: Orientation

CHAPTER 1—HISTORY AND CAREER OPPORTUNITIES IN ESTHETICS

1. c	6. d	11. c
2. a	7. d	12. b
3. d	8. a	13. c
4. c	9. d	14. c
5. b	10. a	15. d

CHAPTER 2—YOUR PROFESSIONAL IMAGE

1. d	6. a	11. d	16. a
2. b	7. a	12. c	17. d
3. a	8. a	13. b	18. c
4. d	9. a	14. a	
5. a	10. a	15. d	

CHAPTER 3—COMMUNICATING FOR SUCCESS

1. a	8. d	15. d	22. d
2. d	9. b	16. d	23. a
3. d	10. a	17. c	24. a
4. a	11. d	18. a	25. d
5. b	12. c	19. b	26. d
6. b	13. d	20. d	
7. d	14. a	21. d	

Part 2: General Sciences

CHAPTER 4—INFECTION CONTROL: PRINCIPLES AND PRACTICE

1. b	9. b	17. a	25. b	33. a
2. a	10. a	18. d	26. b	34. b
3. d	11. b	19. a	27. c	35. b
4. b	12. a	20. b	28. b	36. a
5. a	13. c	21. a	29. a	37. a
6. b	14. b	22. c	30. a	38. a
7. d	15. b	23. a	31. c	
8. a	16. a	24. b	32. a	

CHAPTER 5—GENERAL ANATOMY AND PHYSIOLOGY

1. b	22. a	43. a	64. a
2. d	23. d	44. a	65. a
3. b	24. d	45. d	66. d
4. b	25. a	46. a	67. d
5. c	26. d	47. c	68. b
6. a	27. a	48. d	69. a
7. c	28. b	49. a	70. b
8. b	29. d	50. b	71. a
9. a	30. b	51. b	72. b
10. b	31. b	52. c	73. c
11. c	32. a	53. a	74. a
12. b	33. b	54. c	75. d
13. b	34. a	55. b	76. b
14. a	35. d	56. b	77. d
15. a	36. c	57. d	78. d
16. a	37. d	58. d	79. d
17. b	38. b	59. c	80. a
18. a	39. d	60. a	81. a
19. c	40. d	61. a	82. d
20. d	41. d	62. d	83. b
21. a	42. b	63. a	

CHAPTER 6—BASICS OF CHEMISTRY

1. c	10. c	19. b	28. a
2. a	11. b	20. d	29. d
3. b	12. a	21. c	30. b
4. c	13. d	22. a	31. c
5. c	14. b	23. a	32. a
6. a	15. a	24. a	33. a
7. a	16. d	25. a	34. c
8. c	17. a	26. d	
9. a	18. c	27. a	

CHAPTER 7—BASICS OF ELECTRICITY

1. a	9. d	17. a	25. c
2. c	10. a	18. a	26. a
3. d	11. c	19. b	27. a
4. a	12. d	20. d	28. c
5. c	13. d	21. b	29. d
6. d	14. c	22. c	30. b
7. a	15. a	23. a	31. d
8. d	16. c	24. a	32. a

CHAPTER 8—BASICS OF NUTRITION

1. b	13. c	25. d	37. a
2. a	14. a	26. d	38. a
3. d	15. d	27. a	39. d
4. a	16. a	28. d	40. b
5. a	17. c	29. a	41. a
6. d	18. a	30. a	42. d
7. a	19. b	31. d	43. d
8. c	20. d	32. a	44. b
9. d	21. a	33. d	45. d
10. b	22. b	34. d	
11. a	23. a	35. d	
12. a	24. c	36. c	

Part 3: Skin Sciences

CHAPTER 9—PHYSIOLOGY AND HISTOLOGY OF THE SKIN

1. a	14. a	27. a	40. a
2. d	15. d	28. a	41. a
3. b	16. a	29. a	42. a
4. a	17. c	30. c	43. d
5. c	18. a	31. c	44. a
6. d	19. d	32. b	45. a
7. c	20. b	33. b	46. d
8. b	21. a	34. d	47. c
9. d	22. d	35. d	48. a
10. d	23. a	36. b	49. d
11. a	24. c	37. c	50. a
12. c	25. a	38. a	51. d
13. b	26. d	39. d	

CHAPTER 10—DISORDERS AND DISEASES OF THE SKIN

1. d	13. d	25. a	37. c	49. d
2. b	14. c	26. b	38. d	50. a
3. c	15. d	27. a	39. d	51. b
4. a	16. a	28. d	40. a	52. a
5. c	17. a	29. a	41. d	53. a
6. a	18. b	30. c	42. c	54. d
7. a	19. c	31. d	43. b	55. a
8. d	20. d	32. c	44. a	56. c
9. b	21. a	33. d	45. a	57. d
10. d	22. c	34. b	46. c	
11. c	23. b	35. a	47. d	
12. a	24. d	36. a	48. c	

CHAPTER 11—SKIN ANALYSIS

1. a	11. a	21. a	31. a	41. c
2. a	12. c	22. c	32. c	42. b
3. c	13. d	23. a	33. b	43. c
4. b	14. a	24. d	34. a	44. a
5. c	15. d	25. b	35. d	45. d
6. d	16. c	26. a	36. a	46. a
7. a	17. c	27. c	37. d	47. a
8. d	18. a	28. d	38. a	48. c
9. a	19. b	29. b	39. a	49. d
10. d	20. c	30. d	40. d	

CHAPTER 12—SKIN CARE PRODUCTS: CHEMISTRY, INGREDIENTS, AND SELECTION

1. a	16. a	31. b	46. b	61. d
2. c	17. d	32. a	47. d	62. c
3. d	18. c	33. c	48. d	63. b
4. b	19. d	34. c	49. d	64. d
5. a	20. b	35. a	50. b	65. b
6. c	21. d	36. d	51. a	66. d
7. a	22. d	37. a	52. b	67. c
8. a	23. c	38. b	53. d	68. b
9. d	24. d	39. c	54. b	69. b
10. d	25. a	40. a	55. d	70. d
11. c	26. d	41. d	56. d	71. a
12. a	27. d	42. a	57. c	72. d
13. a	28. a	43. b	58. a	73. c
14. d	29. d	44. a	59. d	
15. c	30. c	45. a	60. a	

Part 4: Esthetics

CHAPTER 13—THE TREATMENT ROOM

1. a	11. d	21. c
2. b	12. a	22. a
3. d	13. b	23. b
4. b	14. c	24. a
5. b	15. a	25. b
6. b	16. d	26. a
7. d	17. d	27. c
8. b	18. d	28. a
9. d	19. a	29. c
10. a	20. b	

CHAPTER 14—BASIC FACIALS

1. b	16. a	31. a
2. a	17. d	32. d
3. c	18. d	33. b
4. d	19. a	34. d
5. d	20. d	35. c
6. d	21. c	36. a
7. a	22. b	37. b
8. b	23. a	38. a
9. a	24. a	39. a
10. b	25. b	40. d
11. a	26. b	41. d
12. d	27. a	42. b
13. a	28. b	43. c
14. a	29. a	44. b
15. b	30. d	45. b

CHAPTER 15—FACIAL MASSAGE

1. d	9. d	17. a
2. b	10. a	18. b
3. d	11. c	19. b
4. a	12. b	20. d
5. c	13. d	21. d
6. a	14. b	22. a
7. d	15. d	23. a
8. b	16. b	24. d

CHAPTER 16—FACIAL MACHINES

1. a	15. d	29. d
2. d	16. d	30. a
3. d	17. b	31. a
4. d	18. d	32. b
5. b	19. b	33. a
6. d	20. b	34. d
7. c	21. a	35. c
8. a	22. b	36. d
9. c	23. d	37. d
10. b	24. a	38. b
11. d	25. d	39. b
12. d	26. b	40. b
13. d	27. a	41. b
14. b	28. a	

CHAPTER 17—HAIR REMOVAL

1. c	14. b	27. d	40. a
2. d	15. c	28. a	41. c
3. b	16. a	29. b	42. a
4. d	17. d	30. a	43. d
5. d	18. b	31. b	44. b
6. c	19. d	32. c	45. c
7. a	20. b	33. a	46. b
8. d	21. a	34. a	47. a
9. b	22. a	35. d	48. a
10. a	23. d	36. a	49. a
11. a	24. a	37. a	50. b
12. b	25. b	38. d	
13. c	26. d	39. a	

CHAPTER 18—ADVANCED TOPICS AND TREATMENTS

1. a	13. c	25. d	37. d
2. d	14. a	26. d	38. a
3. d	15. b	27. a	39. b
4. a	16. c	28. a	40. c
5. d	17. a	29. d	41. d
6. d	18. d	30. d	42. a
7. a	19. a	31. d	43. c
8. b	20. a	32. a	44. d
9. b	21. d	33. d	45. b
10. c	22. d	34. b	46. d
11. d	23. d	35. c	
12. a	24. a	36. b	

CHAPTER 19—THE WORLD OF MAKEUP

1. d	16. b	31. a	46. d	61. a
2. d	17. b	32. b	47. d	62. d
3. d	18. a	33. c	48. a	63. c
4. a	19. d	34. b	49. b	64. a
5. b	20. c	35. a	50. d	65. b
6. c	21. a	36. c	51. d	66. a
7. c	22. b	37. b	52. b	67. b
8. d	23. d	38. b	53. c	68. c
9. a	24. d	39. a	54. a	69. d
10. b	25. a	40. b	55. d	70. d
11. c	26. d	41. a	56. b	71. a
12. d	27. a	42. b	57. c	
13. a	28. b	43. d	58. d	
14. c	29. a	44. d	59. b	
15. d	30. d	45. a	60. c	

Part 5: Business Skills

CHAPTER 20—CAREER PLANNING

1. b	11. d	21. d
2. a	12. a	22. a
3. d	13. b	23. d
4. a	14. c	24. a
5. b	15. d	25. a
6. a	16. a	26. b
7. d	17. d	27. d
8. c	18. c	28. b
9. b	19. a	
10. a	20. a	

CHAPTER 21—THE SKIN CARE BUSINESS

1. d	11. d	21. a
2. c	12. c	22. d
3. a	13. b	23. d
4. a	14. c	24. d
5. c	15. b	25. a
6. b	16. a	26. a
7. c	17. a	27. a
8. a	18. a	28. a
9. d	19. b	29. d
10. c	20. a	

CHAPTER 22—SELLING PRODUCTS AND SERVICES

1. b	7. c	13. b
2. b	8. a	14. d
3. b	9. d	15. b
4. a	10. a	16. c
5. a	11. c	17. b
6. d	12. d	

NOTES

NOTES

NOTES